OXYGEN HEALING THERAPIES

OXYGEN HEALING THERAPIES

FOR OPTIMUM HEALTH & VITALITY
BIO-OXIDATIVE THERAPIES FOR TREATING
IMMUNE DISORDERS · CANDIDA · CANCER ·
HEART, SKIN, CIRCULATORY & OTHER MODERN DISEASES

NATHANIEL ALTMAN

Foreword by
Charles H. Farr, M.D., Ph.D.

Healing Arts Press
Rochester, Vermont

Healing Arts Press
One Park Street
Rochester, Vermont 05767
www.InnerTraditions.com

This revised and expanded edition published by Healing Arts Press in 1998
Copyright © 1995, 1998 by Nathaniel Altman

Note to the reader: *This book is intended as an informational guide.
The remedies, approaches, and techniques described herein are
meant to supplement, and not to be a substitute for, professional
medical care or treatment. They should not be used to treat a serious
ailment without prior consultation with a qualified health-care
professional.*

LIBRARY OF CONGRESS CATALOGING-IN-PUBLICATION DATA

Altman, Nathaniel, 1948–
    Oxygen healing therapies : for optimum health & vitality : bio-oxidative
    therapies for treating immune disorders, candida, cancer, heart, skin,
    circulatory & other modern diseases / Nathaniel Altman ; foreword by
    Charles H. Farr. — Rev. & expanded ed.
        p.   cm.
    Includes bibliographical references and index.
    ISBN 0-89281-793-3 (pbk. : alk. paper)
    1. Hydrogen peroxide—Therapeutic use.   2. Ozone—Therapeutic use.
I. Title.
    RM666.H83A45 1998   98-23505
    6125'.2721—dc21   CIP

Printed and bound in Canada

10 9 8 7 6 5 4 3 2 1

Text design by Charlotte Tyler and Bonnie Atwater
Typesetting and layout by Sarah Albert
This book was set in Optima with OptiBankGothic and OptiAmvet as display
fonts

Healing Arts Press is a division of Inner Traditions International

*This book is dedicated
to the memory of
Adelson de Barros*

Disclaimer

The author of this book is not a physician. The following material is presented in the spirit of historical, philosophical, and scientific inquiry and is *not* offered as medical advice, diagnosis, or treatment of any kind.

Although studies have attested to the safety of bio-oxidative therapies at established therapeutic dose levels, it should be remembered that ozone and hydrogen peroxide are powerful oxidizers. They can be dangerous if not stored, handled, and utilized properly. Oxidizers like food-grade hydrogen peroxide should always be correctly labeled and kept out of reach of children. The author and publisher advise against self-treatment with bio-oxidative therapies. Any medical treatment should be done under the supervision of a qualified health practitioner.

Contents

FOREWORD

This intelligently presented consumer's guide to bio-oxidative therapies will stimulate worldwide appreciation for the therapeutic benefits of ozone and hydrogen peroxide. Much of the data found in this book is being seen for the first time by the vast majority of medical professionals as well as health-care consumers. The evidence shows that millions of people can now be treated effectively for a multitude of illnesses that were considered to be untreatable. When these substances are properly administered, the almost complete lack of adverse side effects places hydrogen peroxide and ozone therapies into a superior class of therapeutic agents never before identified.

The terms used to describe the subject matter in this book—oxygen, ozone, hydrogen peroxide, antioxidants, free radicals—can be confusing. Words like "oxidation" and "oxygenation" are used to describe certain chemical events in reference to oxygen, ozone, or hydrogen peroxide, which sometimes defy understanding by even the best of biochemists. To see how confusing it can be, let us take the words *bio-oxidative therapy*, used as the central theme of this book.

Bio properly refers to the biological term meaning "life" or "living." The term *oxidative* makes most people think of oxygen. When used together, one might think that they would mean "life-oxygen." However, this is incorrect.

Oxidation (even though it sounds like oxygen) is not the same as oxygenation. Properly used, the term *oxidation* means the "grabbing," "taking up," or "scavenging" of an electron from any chemical molecule that might have one available. *Oxygenation*, on the other hand, is a term signifying an *increase* in the number of oxygen molecules. Many things cause oxidation (Vitamin C is a good example) that do not increase the number of oxygen molecules in a chemical reaction. Oxygen, on the other hand, can cause oxidation while at the same time adding more oxygen molecules. This would properly be called oxygenation.

Living and healing are dependent on chemical balance in the body. Some chemical reactions will progress in one direction, called oxidation. Other chemical reactions go in the opposite direction, known as reduction. All life processes are dependent upon these two reactions being in dynamic balance.

Because of the many external influences around us that exert themselves on these sensitive oxidation and reduction reactions—such as air and water pollution—it is difficult to maintain this balance. There is growing evidence that these external environmental factors can cause the body's oxidative and antioxidant systems to become overwhelmed. The net effect is that the body gradually loses its ability to oxidize properly. A major consequence is a negative effect on the body's immune system and its ability to defend against infections, allergens, toxins, and other environmental agents. This gives us reason to consider the use of oxidizers like hydrogen peroxide and ozone to stimulate the body's oxidative enzyme systems and return the body to balance and health.

When hydrogen peroxide and/or ozone are used as therapeutic agents, it soon becomes obvious that they are useful in treating a wide variety of seemingly unrelated conditions. Since most of us have come to think in terms of "one cause, one disease, one cure," we have difficulty accepting the idea that a broad-scope panacea may have been discovered. Yet the concept that hydrogen peroxide, for example, may indeed be a panacea is not so far-fetched when we begin exploring the role of this substance in body metabolism.

Hydrogen peroxide is manufactured by the body and is maintained at a constant level throughout our life. It is part of a system that helps the body regulate living cell membranes. It is a hormonal regulator, necessary for the body to produce several hormonal substances such as estrogen, progesterone, and thyroxine. It is vital for the regulation of blood sugar and the production of energy in all body cells. Hydrogen peroxide helps regulate certain chemicals to operate the brain and nervous system. It has a stimulatory and regulatory effect on the immune system and may either directly or indirectly kill viruses, bacteria, parasites, yeast, fungi, and a variety of other harmful organisms. Our studies demonstrate a positive metabolic effect of an intravenous infusion of hydrogen peroxide. Its ability to oxidize almost any physiological and pathological substance, in addition to producing increased tissue and cellular oxygen tensions, has proved it to have therapeutic value.

Ozone, since it is reduced to hydrogen peroxide after it enters the body, would produce similar effects. Once the involvement of hydrogen peroxide in human metabolism is better understood, the multitude of effects of bio-oxidative therapies on a wide variety of diseases will be easier to understand.

Many of these discoveries are documented in Nathaniel Altman's book. The evidence he presents should stimulate a new appreciation for the potential therapeutic applications of bio-oxidative therapies. The information presented here will add many new pages to the book of modern medical history.

Charles H. Farr, M.D., Ph.D.
Founder and Medical Director,
International Oxidative Medicine Association
Nominee, Nobel Prize (Medicine) 1993

Preface to the Second Edition

Since 1995 when *Oxygen Healing Therapies* was published, dozens of clinical studies around the world have resulted in an impressive amount of new information about the continued safety and effectiveness of therapeutic ozone and hydrogen peroxide. New developments in administering bio-oxidative therapies have also been introduced, from steam cabinet applications to administering ozone through the ears. At the same time, the introduction of a vast number of nonprescription oxygen therapy-related products—including nutritional supplements, colon cleansers, and skin creams—have proliferated in the marketplace along with oxygenated water and oxygen spas. And several important websites dealing with oxygen therapies have been established on the Internet, making reliable information instantly available to people all over the world.

This revised and updated edition brings these new developments and clinical findings to the reading public. We also include additional graphics and charts illustrating some of the new and exciting applications of ozone therapy, as well as an expanded resources section.

I would like to thank several people who assisted me in preparing this new edition. In addition to suggesting changes in the original text, Zdenek (Den) Rasplicka of Ozone Services provided much new information and graphics and Dr. Guy Savoie offered suggestions and information about his personal experiences with ozone. Thanks also go to Brian McAllister for his sound overall advice as well as his practical instruction in the art of ozone applications.

ACKNOWLEDGMENTS

I would like to thank the following people who assisted in the creation of this book by providing information, reviewing the chapters, helping me make contact with other sources of information, and offering advice and encouragement:

Michael Carpendale, M.D.; Silvia Menéndez Cepero, Ph.D.; Geoffrey Rogers; Toby Freedman, M.D.; Alison Johnson; Mildred Aissen; Hilton Santos; Gerard Sunnen, M.D.; Stuart Rynsburger, D.C.; Michael E. Shannon, M.D.; Carlos Hernández Castro, Ph.D.; Siegfried Rilling, M.D.; Horst Kief, M.D.; Jon Greenberg, M.D.; Dr. Juliane Sacher; Lilya Zevin; John C. Pittman, M.D.; and Frank Shallenberger, M.D., H.M.D.

Special thanks go to Siegfried Rilling, M.D., and Haug Publishers for permission to reproduce graphics from the book *The Use of Ozone in Medicine*; to Horst Kief, M.D., for permission to use his photographs of patients; to Charles H. Farr, M.D., Ph.D., for permission to use his chart on the effects of hydrogen peroxide on Shanghai influenza; to Mark Konlee for permission to use material from his book *AIDS Control Diet*; and to Dr. Juliane Sacher for permission to reproduce the information found in her article on vitamin and mineral supplementation.

Acknowledgment is also made to my publisher, Healing Arts Press, for having the courage to be the first in the world to publish a book on bio-oxidative therapies for the general reader.

I would also like to acknowledge those who have worked tirelessly to help make bio-oxidative therapies known to the public, including Ed

McCabe, Geoffrey Rogers, Gary Null, Walter Grotz, Conrad LeBeau, and the late Father Richard Wilhelm. I wish to acknowledge the special role of José Alberto Rosa, M.D., who led me to seriously investigate bio-oxidative therapies.

Special recognition should be given to Drs. Silvia Menéndez Cepero and Manuel Gómez Moraleda for having created and guided the direction of the Centro de Ozono in Cuba. They deserve credit for having been leading proponents for scientific research in ozone and its practical application. Their efforts have had a tremendous impact on the lives of thousands.

Finally, I thank Dr. Charles H. Farr for offering material, reviewing the manuscript, and generously providing the foreword to this book.

INTRODUCTION

My personal interest in bio-oxidative therapies is the result of having been the primary caregiver for a friend with very advanced AIDS who was sent home from the hospital to die.

During the final weeks of his life, I administered daily infusions of diluted 35 percent food-grade hydrogen peroxide under a physician's supervision. To my surprise, it was one of the only therapies that seemed to help. Although my friend did not survive, we were impressed at how the infusions gave him energy, inner peace, and optimism. He experienced far less discomfort than he had before the infusions began and was able to sleep better, as well. He also applied undiluted hydrogen peroxide directly to a Karposi sarcoma lesion on his foot, and it had shrunk by half within three weeks.

Having been interested in complementary and natural therapies for over twenty years, I became intrigued with the healing potential of hydrogen peroxide: If it could make such a difference in the quality of life of a person dying from AIDS-related diseases, how could it help people who were not at death's door?

Ozone—another bio-oxidative therapy—has been used extensively in Europe for over thirty years to treat a wide variety of medical conditions, including heart disease, cancer, and AIDS. However, medical doctors in the United States and Canada who use bio-oxidative therapies are often persecuted by state medical authorities and medical societies. Some have even had their practices closed down.

Now, here was a natural substance that could have a major impact on one's health and was inexpensive, safe, and easy to administer. Thousands of practitioners use it in Europe on millions of patients, but it is often illegal to use here. In fact, hundreds of people leave the United States and Canada every year to receive these therapies elsewhere. They pay for them out of their own pockets, since insurance won't cover "experimental" treatments. At the same time, the mainstream press ignores bio-oxidative therapies completely, and (until now) the only books on the subject were published by the authors themselves.

I soon began reading what I could about hydrogen peroxide and ozone. I also attended an International Bio-Oxidative Medicine Foundation (now the International Oxidative Medicine Association) conference, where I participated in workshops, attended presentations, and reviewed the medical literature offered by dozens of physicians, chemists, and other researchers.

Although I have been writing about holistic and alternative healing for over twenty years, I had not come across any information about bio-oxidative therapies until the late stages of my friend's illness. Several self-published books were available and a number of people like Ed McCabe, Gary Null, and Walter Grotz had been struggling to educate the public for years, but many others (including myself) had never heard about these therapies.

I also learned to my surprise that a tremendous volume of scientific and medical literature on the medical use of ozone and hydrogen peroxide had been published over the past sixty years. Although a few articles were published in well-known journals like *Science, Cancer,* and *The Lancet,* most were published in obscure scientific journals that are rarely read by the general public. I soon realized that there was much more to learn about ozone and hydrogen peroxide, especially in their possible application in areas of preventive health care. I learned that some of the most exciting work in the field of medical ozone therapy is being done in Russia and Cuba but that little information was known outside those countries.

I decided that an objective, scientifically documented yet readable book was needed for the lay reader. I have always believed that information is vital to enable us to make intelligent decisions about our health, and I wanted to assemble the latest and most reliable information about bio-oxidative therapies: what they are, how they work, and what they can do to promote the healing process. I also wanted to introduce these therapies as part of a holistic approach to health, in which body cleansing, diet, and exercise could enhance the therapeutic qualities of hydrogen peroxide and ozone.

Writing this book has been an incredible experience. My research has taken me to Germany and Cuba, and I have met with scientists from Russia, France, and throughout the United States, many of whom have contributed material to this book. I have read hundreds of articles and have spoken to many patients who have received bio-oxidative therapies.

I have been astonished, although not surprised, at the continued opposition of the United States medical authorities and the government toward researching these therapies, let alone allowing their use under medical supervision. While not always a "miracle cure," the proven safety, effectiveness, and medical applications of hydrogen peroxide and ozone warrant far more attention than they have been receiving from the press and the medical and scientific communities in this country. The fact that they are nonpatentable, inexpensive, and useful in the treatment of dozens of diseases plays a primary role in this situation. Unlike expensive pharmaceuticals, surgery, and other advanced medical modalities, these simple therapies are not going to fill the pockets of physicians, drug companies, medical equipment manufacturers, insurance companies, and hospitals. Since those interests—primarily through professional, trade, and political action organizations—influence the direction of health care policy in this country, future research in bio-oxidative therapies will probably not be initiated by them.

The future of alternative therapies like ozone and hydrogen peroxide is in the hands of the health-care consumer in this country, and about 50 percent of us consulted alternative practitioners during a recent year. We support the health-care industry through taxes and by purchasing its products and services. We should demand to have the freedom to choose the healing modalities that we want for ourselves and our families without having such personal decisions made by others.

The purpose of this book is not to persuade anyone to use ozone or hydrogen peroxide. Rather, it is to present the facts about these therapies and show how they are being used in clinics and hospitals throughout the world. It is hoped that this book will stimulate discussion and perhaps eventually lead both the public and the medical and scientific communities to take a more serious look at the therapeutic potential of hydrogen peroxide and ozone. As a result, consumers can make more educated and intelligent decisions regarding our health-care options.

PART I

FOUNDATIONS

In an age of increasing medical specialization, complex and sometimes questionable medical procedures, and expensive, often ineffective medications, many health-care consumers are interested in getting back to basics. They are looking for safe and effective medical therapies that will naturally enhance their innate healing powers. They are looking for therapies that cause a minimum of negative side effects and will not bring about financial ruin.

Most of us feel that such therapies are nonexistent. However, there are two simple, natural substances whose clinical use has been documented in medical literature. Physicians who have used them in this country have been threatened, harassed, and persecuted by state medical associations and the federal government, despite the fact that these substances have been proved effective in treating some of our most common serious diseases including heart disease, cancer, and AIDS. Overlooked by the mainstream medical professions, ignored by the government, and feared by the pharmaceutical industry, they are now being used by a rapidly growing underground of health-care consumers. A small number of physicians who are tired of the expensive, dangerous, invasive, and often useless medical procedures used to treat these diseases are also turning to these substances. The elements are hydrogen peroxide and ozone, used in a therapeutic approach known as *bio-oxidative therapy*.

Bio-oxidative therapies have been used for over 100 years and first appeared in mainstream medical journals in 1920. Since that time, they have been studied in many major medical research centers throughout the world. The foremost American researcher of bio-oxidative therapies, Dr. Charles H. Farr, was nominated for the Nobel Prize in Medicine in 1993 for his work.

Hydrogen peroxide is involved in all of life's vital processes and must be present for the immune system to function properly. The cells in the body that fight infection (know as granulocytes) produce hydrogen peroxide as a first line of defense against invading organisms like parasites, viruses, bacteria, and yeast. It is also required for the metabolism of protein, carbohydrates, fats, vitamins, and minerals. As a hormonal regulator, hydrogen peroxide is necessary for the body's production of estrogen, progesterone, and thyroxin. It also helps regulate blood sugar and the production of energy in cells. Hydrogen peroxide has long been known medically as a disinfectant, antiseptic, and oxidizer. Recently it has been used to successfully treat a wide variety of human diseases—including circulatory disorders, pulmonary diseases, parasitic infections, and immune-related disorders—with few harmful side effects.

Ozone is an energized form of oxygen with extra electrons and was originally used to disinfect wounds during World War I. It was later found that ozone can "blast" holes through the membranes of viruses, yeasts, bacteria, and abnormal tissue cells before killing them. Ozone was the focus of considerable research during the 1930s in Germany, where it was successfully used to treat patients suffering from inflammatory bowel disorders, ulcerative colitis, Crohn's disease, and chronic bacterial diarrhea. There is evidence that ozone can destroy many viruses, including those related to hepatitis, Epstein–Barr, cancer, herpes, cytomegalovirus, and HIV.

Recently, the United States government (through the Office of Alternative Medicine at the National Institutes of Health) has become more receptive to the idea of bio-oxidative therapies. It is hoped that human trials will begin as additional clinical data are presented to this office (especially data regarding complete remission of AIDS symptoms and seronegative tests for HIV-positive patients).

Hydrogen peroxide and ozone hold great promise in helping to treat some of the most devastating diseases confronting humanity today. Together, they form the "cutting edge" of a new healing paradigm involving safe, effective, natural, and inexpensive forms of medical therapy.

In the following section, we introduce bio-oxidative therapies and examine their theoretical basis.

7

1

WHAT ARE BIO-OXIDATIVE
THERAPIES?

Oxygen is essential for life. As the most abundant element of the Earth's crust, oxygen compounds form a major part of oceans, rocks, and all other living things. In fact, over 62 percent of the Earth's crust (by mass) is made up of oxygen. It also constitutes 65 percent of the elements of our body, including blood, organs, tissues, and skin.[1]

Oxygen is a clear, odorless gas that can easily be dissolved in water. Each molecule of oxygen (a molecule being the smallest amount of a chemical substance that can exist by itself without changing or breaking apart) is composed of two atoms of oxygen and is known by the chemical formula O_2.

Oxygen is involved with all body functions, and we require a continual supply of oxygen to survive. The average person needs some 200 milliliters (about 1 cup) of oxygen per minute while resting and nearly 8 liters (approximately 2 gallons) during periods of strenuous activity. The brain—which makes up about 2 percent of our total body mass—requires over 20 percent of the body's oxygen needs. While we can go without food for several months and survive without water for a couple of days, we cannot live without oxygen for more than a few minutes.

Oxygen makes up 21 percent of the air we normally breathe.* Smokers or people who live in heavily polluted environments are likely to consume less. The oxygen we breathe reacts with sugars (from the food

* The other principal component of air is nitrogen: Air consists of four volumes of nitrogen to one of oxygen.

8

we eat and from the breakdown of fats and starch in the body) to produce carbon dioxide, water, and energy. The energy from this process, a form of combustion, is stored in a compound called adenosine triphosphate (ATP). ATP is essentially the fuel we use to live, think, and move. According to Sheldon Saul Hendler, M.D., in his book *The Oxygen Breakthrough*, oxygen is the most vital component of ATP within our cells:

> ATP is the basic currency of life. Without it, we are literally dead. Imbalance or interruption in the production and flow of this substance results in fatigue, disease and disorder, including immune imbalance, cancer, heart disease and all of the degenerative processes we associate with aging.[2]

The lungs, heart, and circulatory system deliver sufficient amounts of oxygen to the entire body. This oxygen creates the energy we need to survive and thrive. At the same time, the lungs take the waste product carbon dioxide (CO_2) from the blood and discharge it back into the air. It is estimated that we breathe in 2500 gallons of air each day. In contrast, trees take in carbon dioxide and, through the process of photosynthesis, convert carbon dioxide into oxygen and send it back into the atmosphere for us to enjoy once more.

We all know how tired and sluggish we feel when we are in a closed room full of people. Although the room is filled with air, that air is high in carbon dioxide and deficient in oxygen. A number of studies have linked the high CO_2 level in the cabins of commercial jet aircraft (which is almost double the minimum comfort standard for indoor air) to a variety of temporary health problems, including headaches, exhaustion, and eye, nose, and throat discomfort.[3] When passengers leave the aircraft and oxygen consumption returns to normal, symptoms often disappear within a couple of hours.

Oxygen is absolutely essential for healthy cells, and it acts against toxins in the body. Many pathogens are *anaerobic*, meaning that they thrive in a low-oxygen environment. Cancer cells are among those that are anaerobic. In 1966, Nobel Prize winner Dr. Otto Warburg confirmed that the key precondition for the development of cancer is a lack of oxygen on the cellular level.[4]

How Do Humans Become Oxygen Deficient?

Polluted Air

Perhaps the most important factor in oxygen deficiency is air pollution. For those who smoke or are unfortunate enough to breathe in second-hand smoke, the oxygen content of the air is even lower. Automobile exhaust, factory emissions, and burning garbage are the three greatest causes of lowered oxygen content in the air we breathe.

Devitalized Foods

As we show later, fresh fruits and vegetables contain an abundance of oxygen that is dissolved in water. When we eat generous amounts of fresh, raw vegetables and fruits, our intake of oxygen is increased along with the valuable vitamins and minerals these foods contain.

Foods that have been heavily processed, cooked, and preserved through canning tend to be very low in oxygen. High-fat foods like meat, eggs, and dairy products tend to be lower in oxygen as well. The standard American diet tends to be very low in oxygen content. It should be no surprise that that type of diet has been linked to a wide variety of degenerative diseases like atherosclerosis, cancer, and diabetes.

Poor Breathing

Healthy breathing involves deep, rhythmic breaths that fill the lungs with air and then exhale that air fully back into the atmosphere. Because of pollution, stress, or simply habit, most people do not breathe fully. For example, many of us were taught to breathe by relying on the muscles of the upper chest only, which tends to ventilate the upper part of the lungs only. By utilizing the diaphragm as well as the upper chest in breathing, we are able to take fuller breaths and utilize more of the available oxygen in the lungs. We'll examine the subject of breathing later on.

Oxidation

The primary effect that breathing has on the body is *oxidation*. Oxidation is a natural process that involves oxygen combining with another substance. As a result, the chemical composition of both substances changes. Technically speaking, oxidation includes any reactions in which electrons (tiny particles smaller than an atom that have an electrical charge) are transferred. Most oxidations produce large amounts of energy as light, heat, or electricity. The products of oxidation include corrosion, decay, burning, and respiration.[5] By exposing certain metals to oxygen, for example, the metal is oxidized, producing rust. When butter is left out in the open air for long periods of time, the process of oxidation turns the butter rancid.

Oxidation is also a primary component of combustion. When we light a fire in the fireplace, we are causing the wood to become oxidized. When we start our car engine in the morning, gasoline combines with oxygen and is oxidized to water and carbon dioxide.

Oxidation occurs as combustion within the body when oxygen turns sugar into energy. Our body also uses oxidation and oxidation products as its first line of defense against harmful bacteria, viruses, yeasts, and parasites. Oxidizing molecules attack the pathogenic cells, and they are removed from the body through its normal processes of elimination.

After oxidation, the most important effect of breathing is *oxygenation.* Oxygenation involves saturation with oxygen, as in the aeration of blood in the lungs. Breathing in oxygen is a major source of oxygenation. While hydrogen peroxide and ozone are best known as oxidizers, they are powerful oxygenators as well.

If the oxygenation process within the body is weak or deficient, the body cannot eliminate poisons adequately, and a toxic reaction can occur. In minor cases, a toxic buildup can lead to fatigue, dullness, and sluggishness. However, when poor oxygenation is chronic, our overall immune response to germs and viruses is weakened, making us vulnerable to a wide range of diseases.

Oxidation and Free-Radical Production

One of the medical establishment's chief reservations about the use of oxidants like ozone and hydrogen peroxide in medicine is the production of *free radicals.* A free radical has been defined as "any molecule that possesses an unpaired electron, an electrically-charged particle spinning in lonely orbit and searching for another electron to counterbalance it."[6]

Stable molecules have electrons in pairs. To become stable, a free radical will steal an electron from a stable molecule, which then becomes a free radical itself. Free-radical formation follows a chain reaction, with one free radical causing important structural changes in many other molecules. Cell damage, including mutations, often results.

Yet, free radicals are not necessarily "bad." In fact, many are essential to life. Free radicals (including superoxide and hydroxyl radicals) are produced by the body to deliver energy to the body's cells. In addition, free radicals are used to kill bacteria, fungi, and viruses. For example, when we are exposed to a flu virus, free radicals are formed to destroy it. Free radicals also play an important role in regulating the chemicals the body needs for its survival, such as hormones.

Free radicals are manufactured by the body (they are produced in extra-high amounts during vigorous exercise, but people who are in good physical shape are easily able to detoxify them) and are formed by certain medications. Free radicals are also formed in the environment. Air pollution (including ozone-laden smog, automobile exhaust, and tobacco smoke), toxic wastes, certain food additives, pesticide residues, and radiation (such as radiation from X rays and airplane travel) all produce free radicals that can affect us in different ways.

When we have too many free radicals in our bodies, cell damage can occur. In his book *Free Radicals and Disease Prevention*, David Lin lists how excess free radicals can cause harmful effects to cells; they can

- break off the membrane proteins, destroying a cell's identity

- fuse together membrane lipids (fats) and membrane proteins, hardening the cell membrane and making it brittle

- puncture the cell membrane, allowing bacteria and viruses easy entrance

- disrupt the nuclear membrane, opening up the nucleus and exposing genetic material

- mutate and destroy genetic material, rewriting and destroying genetic information

- burden the immune system with the above havoc and threaten the immune system itself by undermining immune cells with similar damage[7]

As a result, free-radical damage has been linked to a number of degenerative diseases, including atherosclerosis, cancer, cataracts, diabetes, allergies, mental disorders, and arthritis. Excess free radicals also play a role in the aging process and decreased immune response, opening the door to a variety of immune disorders, including the onset of AIDS.[8]

Antioxidants

For the most part, the body regulates the excessive production of free radicals. It does so by producing *antioxidants*. Antioxidants are enzymes (such as catalase, superoxide dismutase, and glutathione peroxidase) that protect cells from free radicals by chemically changing them into harmless compounds like oxygen and water.

In their book *Antioxidant Adaptation*, Stephen A. Levine, Ph.D., and Parris M. Kidd, Ph.D., wrote about the ability of the body's antioxidant defense system to fight off free-radical attacks by providing greater tolerance to oxidative stress to selected tissues:

> The system is flexible: individual antioxidant factors can interact to donate electrons on to another, thereby facilitating the regeneration of optimally active (fully-reduced) forces. The system is also versatile and can respond adaptively to abnormal oxidative challenges subject to source and site availability of required factors. . . . The adaptability of the antioxidant defense system appears to be rather remarkable.[9]

Nutritional Antioxidants

Because excess free-radical activity can seriously deplete our body's natural antioxidant reserves, nutritionists recommend that we augment those supplies with foods rich in antioxidants. Three common vitamins—beta carotene (vitamin A), vitamin C, and vitamin E—are important antioxidants, as are minerals like zinc and selenium. According to Natalie Angier, writing in *The New York Times Magazine*:

> Vitamin E and beta carotene both are used in the fatty membranes of the cell, sponging up free radicals before the vagrants can poke holes into the cellular sheath. Vitamin C, a water soluble compound, works in the

13

aqueous innards of the cell, coupling with radicals and allowing them to be flushed away in the urine.[10]

Many of the foods we eat—green and yellow vegetables, fruits, nuts, and seeds—contain antioxidant vitamins and minerals in abundance and are recommended as a major part of all healthy diets. Many people take nutritional supplements rich in antioxidants for additional protection. The role of nutrition as an adjunct to bio-oxidative therapy is discussed in chapters 9 and 10.

Bio-oxidative Therapies

We mentioned earlier that a major part of free-radical activity involves oxidizing the pathogenic by-products of modern living, which result from environmental pollution, stress, and radiation. A growing number of physicians believe that if the body's antioxidant requirements are met, adding certain oxidative substances to the body is safe as long as those substances are of the right kind and are introduced in the proper manner. Utilizing the principles of oxidation to bring about improvements in the body is known as *bio-oxidative therapy.* This term was first introduced in 1986 by Dr. C. H. Farr in his monograph *The Therapeutic Use of Intravenous Hydrogen Peroxide.*

While aerobic-type exercises; deep, rhythmic breathing; and high-oxygen foods (like fresh fruits and vegetables) promote the normal oxidation process in the body, two natural elements—ozone and hydrogen peroxide—are among the most powerful oxidizers available to humanity and form the essence of bio-oxidative therapy today.

The medical potential for bio-oxidative therapies is based on the relationship of oxygen to human cells. Bio-oxidative therapies accelerate oxygen metabolism and stimulate the release of oxygen atoms from the bloodstream to the cells. When levels of oxygen increase, the potential for disease decreases. When large amounts of oxygen flood the body, germs, parasites, fungi, bacteria, and viruses are killed along with diseased and deficient tissue cells. At the same time, healthy cells not only survive but are better able to multiply. The result is a stronger immune system and improved overall immune response.

Although ozone and hydrogen peroxide are highly toxic in their purified states, they have been found to be safe and effective when diluted to therapeutic levels for medical use. When they are administered in prescribed amounts, the chance of experiencing adverse reactions to bio-oxidative therapies is extremely small. For example, a German study evaluating the side effects of over five million medically administered ozone treatments found that the rate of adverse side effects was only 0.0007 per application. This figure is far lower than in any other type of medical therapy.[11]

Although few of us have heard of them, bio-oxidative therapies have been around for a long time. They have been used clinically by European physicians for over a century and were first reported by Dr. I. N. Love in the *Journal of the American Medical Association* in 1888. Since that time, they have been studied in many major medical research centers throughout the world, including those at Baylor University, Yale University, the University of California (Los Angeles), and Harvard University in the United States, as well as medical schools and laboratories in Great Britain, Germany, Russia, Canada, Japan, Cuba, Mexico, and Brazil. Today, between fifty and one hundred scientific articles about the chemical and biological effects of ozone and hydrogen peroxide are published each month.

Hyperbaric Oxygen Therapy

Hyperbaric oxygen (HBO) therapy is a type of oxygen therapy in which 100 percent pure oxygen is administered at two to three times normal atmospheric pressure. In HBO therapy, the patient is placed in a specially designed chamber. The pressure in the chamber is gradually increased, which causes a rise in the body's blood plasma oxygen content. This results in enhanced tissue oxygen delivery to the compromised tissues. With HBO therapy, oxygen can be dissolved in the blood plasma and go directly into tissues. It also has an important systemic effect on bacterial growth and enhances the body's overall inflammatory response. Hyperbaric oxygen reduces swelling or edema in body tissues. It also produces antioxidant effects and promotes new blood vessel formation in areas of the body where blood supply is limited.

Hyperbaric oxygen has been used to treat a wide range of health problems. It is best known as a primary therapy in treating carbon monoxide poisoning, gas gangrene, and tissue decompression, known in scuba diving as the bends. However, hyperbaric oxygen therapy is now increasingly being used as an adjunct to standard medical and surgical care, including the treatment of problem wounds, anaerobic infections, chronic bone infections, gas embolism, crush injuries, soft-tissue injuries, burns, compromised skin grafts, and radiation injuries. It has been found to be useful in treating patients suffering from impaired healing or compromised blood circulation where oxygen cannot reach important tissues.

HBO has also been found useful in treating people with diabetes and vascular disease as well as amputees, cancer patients undergoing radiation therapy, and patients recovering from plastic, cosmetic, or laser surgery. Research is now underway to study the effects of HBO therapy on patients suffering from stroke, HIV-related disorders, and chronic fatigue syndrome.

Hyperbaric oxygen therapy is finding greater acceptance in treating sports injuries and is believed to enhance performance in competitive athletics. Hyperbaric chambers were widely used in the former Soviet Union, East Germany, and other socialist countries. In the West, some of the professional sports teams have hyperbaric chambers in their training rooms, including the Vancouver Canucks. However, large-scale scientific studies on the ability of HBO therapy to enhance athletic performance are yet to be carried out.

A typical treatment lasts between an hour and ninety minutes, and the number of treatments given depends on the patient's medical condition. For example, divers suffering from the bends would normally receive one or two treatments, while an individual with a severe or infected wound may require daily HBO treatments for several weeks.

Hyperbaric oxygen therapy has several general health benefits:

1. It reduces gas embolism. Any free gas trapped in the body will decrease in volume as pressure exerted on it increases. This may allow it to pass through into general blood. This makes HBO especially useful in management of gas embolism and decompression illness among divers.

2. Hyperbaric oxygen causes the blood vessels to contract. This can result in the reduction of healing time for burn or crush injuries. At the same time, HBO therapy provides extra oxygen to the blood plasma, so that a net increase in tissue oxygen occurs. This, in turn, promotes healing.

3. HBO has an anti-ischemic effect on body tissues. Ischemia occurs when the flow of blood is reduced to a part of the body,

which slows the healing process. Hyperbaric oxygen physically dissolves oxygen into plasma. This allows an increase in the quantity of oxygen transferred to the ischemic tissue by the blood, thus promoting healing.

4. Oxygen is a powerful antimicrobial. Anaerobic bacteria (or bacteria that thrive in a low-oxygen environment) do not contain natural defenses to protect them from superoxides, peroxides, and other compounds formed in the presence of high oxygen tension. Many of the body's defense mechanisms are dependent on oxygen, and when tissue PO_2 drops too low, effective infection-fighting mechanisms are retarded. By reoxygenating those body tissues, we allow the body's defense mechanisms to function at an optimum level once more.

5. Oxygen promotes the formation of new blood cells. Our body's defense mechanisms (such as the "oxidative burst") are necessary for the formation of white blood cells, which kill bacteria and produce collagen, a protein that helps heal wounds. When hypoxia (or oxygen starvation) is reversed by HBO therapy, these body processes are enhanced.

Although HBO therapy is worthy of deeper consideration, it will not be included in the scope of our discussion in this book. During their ground-breaking research at Baylor University in Texas during the 1960s, scientists discovered that many of the positive effects of HBO therapy could be reproduced or enhanced through the therapeutic use of hydrogen peroxide, resulting in much lower treatment cost. Similar findings have been discovered with ozone therapy as well, making both therapies easily available in a traditional medical setting and to patients living in developing countries or in other areas where expensive hyperbaric oxygen chambers are rarely found.[13]

How are Bio-oxidative Therapies Used?

In bio-oxidation therapies tiny amounts of ozone or hydrogen peroxide, added to a base of oxygen or water, are used to flood the body with active forms of oxygen by intravenous, oral, intradermal, or rectal means. Once in the body, the ozone or hydrogen peroxide directly and indirectly becomes damaging to viruses, bacteria, fungi, microbes, and diseased and deficient tissue cells. Through oxidation, these disease microorganisms are killed and eliminated from the body. In this way, ozone and hydrogen peroxide act as purifying agents.

It has been estimated that over ten million people (primarily in Germany, Russia, and Cuba) have been given bio-oxidative therapies over the past seventy years to treat over forty different diseases, including heart and blood vessel diseases, diseases of the lungs, infectious diseases, and immune-related disorders. According to the International Oxidative Medicine Association (IOMA), the following conditions or diseases have been treated with ozone and hydrogen peroxide with varying degrees of success. In some cases bio-oxidative therapies are administered alone, while in others they are used in addition to traditional medical procedures (such as surgery or chemotherapy) or as adjuncts to alternative health practices like megavitamin therapy, acupuncture, or herbalogy.

Heart and Blood Vessel Diseases

Cardiac arrhythmias (irregular heartbeat)
Cardioconversion (heart stoppage)
Cardiovascular disease (heart disease)
Cerebral vascular disease (stroke and memory loss)
Coronary spasm (angina)
Gangrene (of fingers and toes)
Peripheral vascular disease (poor circulation)
Raynaud's disease ("white finger")
Temporal arteritis (inflammation of the temporal artery)
Vascular and cluster headaches

Pulmonary Diseases

Asthma
Bronchiectasis (dilatation of bronchus or bronchi)
Chronic bronchitis
Chronic obstructive pulmonary disease
Emphysema
Pneumocystis carinii (PCP or AIDS-related pneumonia)

Infectious Diseases

Acute and chronic viral infections
Chronic unresponsive bacterial infections

Epstein–Barr virus (chronic fatigue syndrome)
Herpes simplex (fever blister)
Herpes zoster (shingles)
HIV-related infections
Influenza
Parasitic infections
Systemic chronic candidiasis (candida)

Immune Disorders

Diabetes mellitus type II
Hypersensitive reactions (environmental and universal reactors)
Multiple sclerosis
Rheumatoid arthritis

Other Diseases

Alzheimer's disease
Cancers of the blood and lymph nodes[14]
Chronic pain syndromes (due to multiple causes)
Migraine headaches
Pain of metastatic carcinoma
Parkinson's disease

How Do Bio-oxidative Therapies Work?

According to Frank Shallenberger, M.D., bio-oxidative therapies have been found to have the following effects on the human body:

1. Bio-oxidative therapies stimulate the production of white blood cells, which are necessary to fight infection.

2. Ozone and hydrogen peroxide are virucidal.

3. Bio-oxidative therapies increase oxygen and hemoglobin disassociation, thus increasing the delivery of oxygen from the blood to the cells.

4. Ozone and hydrogen peroxide are antineoplastic, which means that they inhibit the growth of new tissues like tumors.

5. Bio-oxidative therapies oxidize and degrade petrochemicals.

6. Bio-oxidative therapies increase red blood cell membrane distensibility, thus enhancing their flexibility and effectiveness.

7. Ozone and hydrogen peroxide therapies increase the production of interferon and tumor necrosis factor, which the body uses to fight infections and cancers.

8. Bio-oxidative therapies increase the efficiency of the antioxidant enzyme system, which scavenges excess free radicals in the body.

9. They accelerate the citric acid cycle, which is the main cycle for the liberation of energy from sugars. This then stimulates basic metabolism. It also breaks down proteins, carbohydrates, and fats to be used as energy.

10. Ozone and hydrogen peroxide therapies increase tissue oxygenation, thus bringing about patient improvement.[15]

Unknown, Ignored, and Forgotten

Although both ozone and hydrogen peroxide therapies have been proved in clinical trials (and in regular clinical practice) to be safe and effective in Germany, Cuba, Mexico, Russia, Italy, France, and Australia, few people have heard about bio-oxidative therapies in the United States and Canada. Although an estimated fifteen thousand European practitioners legally use bio-oxidative therapies in their practices, the number of physicians using these therapies in North America is small, partly because information about ozone and hydrogen peroxide is not provided in medical schools. The medical establishment does not advocate the use of bio-oxidative therapies and often discourages or prevents licensed physicians from using them in their medical practices. Because bio-oxidative therapies are considered experiments or "quackery" in the United States, medical doctors have been threatened with having their licenses revoked if they administer hydrogen peroxide or ozone. Clinics have been closed down, and practitioners have been threatened with jail.

Perhaps the best-known victim of government persecution is Robert Atkins, M.D., the well-known author of *Dr. Atkins' Diet Revolution.* As director of the Atkins Center for Complementary Medicine in New York City, Dr. Atkins had his medical license revoked for treating patients with ozone. After regaining his license in court, Dr. Atkins's 1993 lawsuit against New York State brought about the passage of a law permitting physicians to use ozone and other non-FDA-approved modalities. Yet even before the government attempted to take away his license, the FDA harassed him through his supplier of ozone equipment. During an interview with Geoffrey Rogers for the award-winning film *Ozone and the Politics of Medicine,* Dr. Atkins said:

> Well, I had an ozone generator, and we used it on all our AIDS patients, just about [on] all our cancer patients, and we used it on the yeast patients which was really the largest group. Generally we gave it intravenously, [via] autohemotherapy, where we pull the blood out, mix the blood with ozone, and in a few minutes gave ozonated blood back to the patient.
>
> We found that our cancer protocol, which includes ozone, was effective and was keeping people alive, and without ever having to require pain medicine, without losing weight, without any sign of deterioration. And then when we lost our ozone machine, the patients began to go downhill. The FDA saw to it that our manufacturer had to take away the business end of the machine, so we no longer had an effective ozone generating machine. That's where we are . . . currently. I'm right now trying to figure out how to get around that, because I believe that my patients need ozone.[16]

A major reason for the lack of interest in bio-oxidative therapies is that ozone and hydrogen peroxide are nonpatentable substances that are very inexpensive to manufacture and utilize. There are no financial incentives to incorporate them into traditional medical practice.

Typically, bio-oxidative therapies properly administered in a medical setting cost up to 50 percent less than traditional therapies, especially for chronic and degenerative diseases. Ozone and hydrogen peroxide pose a threat to the continued dominance of the medical establishment: the pharmaceutical industry, medical centers, and physicians who are accustomed to prescribing expensive drugs, complex medical procedures, and long hospital stays.

Because United States government agencies like the Food and Drug Administration (FDA) and the National Institutes of Health (NIH) are influenced by the pharmaceutical industry and the medical lobby, objective investigation and development of effective protocols for bio-oxidative therapies have been difficult to undertake. According to Michael T. F. Carpendale, M.D., a pioneer ozone researcher and professor of orthopedic surgery at the University of California School of Medicine:

In the FDA, the drug companies have representatives on nearly all the committees. If there's something which may be very effective but may undersell the average drug company, of course they are not going to be very pleased if it gets developed. It might be very difficult for them to compete with that. And ozone is obviously inexpensive to produce, it is very potent [and] if it works half as well as the Germans claim it does, everyone should be using it.[17]

Dr. Horst Kief, one of the first physicians in the world to successfully treat HIV-infected patients with ozone, commented on why so little government-sponsored and drug company research is taking place regarding ozone therapy: "Nobody in the pharmaceutical industry can sell ozone. That's the main reason. When we can find a way to sell ozone, I am sure that ozone [will be] the most important drug in the world."[18]

By 1998, the drug industry in the United States was estimated to be a $12 billion business, with annual sales expected to reach $168.59 billion by 2002. With an average net profit margin of 16.4 percent, the American pharmaceutical industry is one of the most profitable sectors of all industry groups.[19]

As a powerful economic and political force in the United States and around the world, these giant multinationals play a major role in determining government policy and influencing medical schools (through research grants) and physicians themselves through advertising in medical journals (the January 1994 edition of *Journal of the American Medical Association* contained twenty-five full pages of drug advertisements), sponsorship of conferences and seminars, outright gifts, and free samples of medications.

Given the tremendous influence and power of these companies, it is amazing that bio-oxidative therapies are practiced to even the modest extent that they are. As these inexpensive, nonpatentable, and multi-disease therapies become better known, we can be certain that the pharmaceutical industry will strengthen its resolve to make medical ozone and hydrogen peroxide unavailable to the general public and will continue to lobby to prevent research and clinical application.

The eleven biggest drug companies trading on the New York Stock Exchange reported 1996 sales and profits and 2000–2002 estimates as seen in table 1.1.

Table 1.1 Annual Sales and Profits of America's Largest Drug Companies

Company	Sales (billion dollars)		Net Profits (billion dollars)		Net Profit Margin (percent)
	1996	2000–02 est.	1996	2000–02 est.	2000–02 est.
American Home Products Corp.	14.088	20.360	1.883	3.705	18.2
Bristol-Myers Squibb Co.	15.065	22.200	2.850	4.640	20.9
Eli Lilly & Co.	7.347	13.200	1.458	3.370	25.5
Glaxo Wellcome Plc	13.012	19.500	1.527	2.970	15.2
Merck & Co.	19.829	35.500	3.881	7.100	20.0
Pfizer, Inc.	11.306	18.750	1.929	3.535	18.8
Pharmacia & Upjohn, Inc.	7.176	9.000	977	1.445	16.1
Rhone-Poulenc Rorer	5.421	6.775	474	925	13.7
Schering-Plough, Corp.	5.656	8.900	1.213	2.045	23.0
SmithKline Beecham	13.552	20.475	1.431	2.655	13.0
Warner Lambert Co.	7.231	13.250	694	1.990	15.0

Source: The Value Line Investment Survey, *August 1, 1997, 1238–66.*

2

OZONE

Ozone is an elemental form of oxygen occurring naturally in the Earth's atmosphere. It is created in nature when ultraviolet energy causes oxygen atoms to temporarily recombine in groups of three. Ozone is also formed by the action of electrical discharges on oxygen, so it is often created by thunder and lightning. After a thunderstorm, the air seems to smell like freshly mown hay because of the small quantities of ozone generated by the storm. Ozone is also produced commercially in ozone generators, which send an electrical discharge through a specially built condenser containing oxygen. Figure 2.1 shows the principle behind ozone generation.

Because it is made up of three atoms of oxygen, ozone is known chemically as O_3. The newly formed molecule is quick to react with other substances.

A pale blue gas that condenses to a deep blue liquid at very low temperatures, ozone surrounds the Earth at an altitude of between 50,000 and 100,000 feet.[1] When it occurs in the upper atmosphere, ozone forms a protective layer that absorbs much of the sun's ultraviolet radiation. If it were not for the ozone layer, the survival of animal and plant life on this planet would be impossible. The depletion of the ozone layer by the use of chlorofluorocarbons (CFCs)—released into the atmosphere by refrigerators, air conditioners, and aerosol containers—has become a grave concern to scientists and physicians the world over. The dangerous ultraviolet light that would ordinarily be blocked by the ozone layer has been linked to a wide variety of human health problems, including

Figure 2.1. Principle of ozone generation. (From Siegfried Rilling and Renate Viebahn, The Use of Ozone in Medicine Heidelberg: Haug Publishers, 1987. Reprinted courtesy of Dr. Siegfried Rilling and Haug Publishers.)

skin cancer and immunosuppression. Ultraviolet radiation has also been a factor in poor growth of certain species of grains. After many years of study and much procrastination by industry and government, efforts are finally being made to phase out the use of CFCs completely.

In the lower atmosphere, ozone combines with hydrocarbons (like carbon dioxide) and nitrogen oxide in vehicular exhaust and other sources, creating photochemical smog. As a result, new and often highly corrosive pollutants are formed. The number of possible chemical reactions that can occur when ozone is combined with these oxides can reach into the hundreds. The effects of ozone-laden smog have been linked to acid rain, a variety of lung-related diseases, and the oxidation of buildings and monuments, especially in smoggy cities like Los Angeles, Mexico City, and São Paulo.

Many people believe that ozone is toxic because ozone is associated with these reactions. Yet the ozone index published in the newspapers and announced during the evening weather report is only an assay for estimating how much toxic nitrous oxide and hydrocarbons are present in the atmosphere. As a powerful oxidizer, ozone actually helps clean the atmosphere of hydrogen monoxide, nitrous oxide, sulfur dioxide, and dozens of other dangerous compounds. Rather than warn of the dangers of breathing ozone only, weather reporters should focus more on breathing these other (and far more dangerous) elements of smog, formed primarily by vehicle exhaust and factory emissions.

Scientific studies in this country have emphasized the negative effects of ozone on breathing. That may be one reason physicians and others feel that ozone is not only medically useless but also a dangerous substance to take into the body under any circumstances. However, as we will see, the value of ozone cannot be dismissed so easily.

History

Ozone's distinctive odor was first reported by Van Mauran in 1785, but the gas was not actually "discovered" until 1840 by the German chemist Christian Frederick Schönbein at the University of Basel in Switzerland. He decided to name the gas ozone (from the Greek word for "smell") because of its pungent odor. In 1860, the French chemist Soret concluded that the ozone molecule was made up of three atoms of oxygen. However, it was the English chemist Andrews, a member of the Royal Society of London, who demonstrated many of ozone's oxidating and disinfecting properties for the first time in a laboratory.

In 1856, ozone gas was used for the first time to disinfect operating rooms, and in 1860, the first water treatment plant to use ozone to purify municipal water supplies was built in Monaco. After a severe cholera epidemic in Hamburg killed thirty thousand people, the first waterworks to use ozone in Germany was constructed by the chemist and inventor Werner von Siemens (the company he founded has evolved into the huge German conglomerate that bears his name) in Wiesbaden in 1901, followed by one in the Westphalian city of Paderborn a year later.[2] The process of purifying water with ozone is a simple one: A small amount of ozone is added to oxygen and mixed with the drinking water. Ozone kills viruses and bacteria and removes the micro-organisms that cause bad taste and odor in the water. Today, over a thousand cities around the world use ozone to purify their drinking supplies.

Since the early part of this century, many advances have been made in ozone technology. Sophisticated ozone generators and related technologies that incorporate ozone in a wide range of industrial and scientific applications have been developed. Over the past few years a number of ozone-resistant materials have been developed for use with ozone generators. In addition to custom-blown glass components, modern substances like Teflon, a form of plastic known as PVDF or Kynar, a rubberlike substance called Viton, and silicone for flexible tubing are becoming increasingly available.

Medical Ozone

After the turn of the century, interest began to focus on the uses of ozone in medical therapy. The Berlin physician Albert Wolff first utilized ozone to treat skin diseases in 1915, and the German army used ozone extensively during World War I to treat a wide variety of battle wounds and anaerobic infections.

It was not until 1932, however, that ozone was seriously studied by the scientific community. Ozonated water was used as a disinfectant by Dr. E. A. Fisch, a German dentist. One of his patients was the surgeon Erwin Payr, who immediately saw the possibilities of ozone in medical therapy. Dr. Payr, along with the French physician P. Aubourg, was the first medical doctor to apply ozone gas through rectal insufflation to treat mucous colitis and fistulae. In 1945, Payr pioneered the method of injecting ozone intravenously for the treatment of circulatory disturbances.

Other German pioneers in medical ozone included the physicist Joaquim Hansler, who developed the first medical ozone generator that could make accurate dosages of oxygen and ozone. The company he founded, which bears his name, is now the largest manufacturer of medical ozone generators in the world. Figure 2.2 shows the latest in

Figure 2.2. Portable medical ozone generator. (Photo courtesy of Kastner Praxisbedarf GmbH-Medizintechnik, Rastatt, Germany.)

portable medical ozone generators from Germany, while a larger generator for hospital use can be seen in figure 2.3 (see page 40).

The Second World War brought about major setbacks for German research into medical ozone, as many clinics and laboratories were destroyed in Allied air raids. It was not until the 1950s that clinics reopened and research began again.

The first physician to treat cancer with ozone was Dr. W. Zable in the late 1950s, followed by Drs. P. G. Seeger, A. Varro, and H. Werkmeister. During the next twenty years, hundreds of German physicians began using ozone in their practices (both alone and as a complement to traditional medical therapy) to treat a wide variety of diseases through a number of applications. Horst Kief is believed to have been the first doctor to use ozone therapy to successfully treat patients infected with the human immunodeficiency virus (HIV). He also pioneered the development of autohomologous immunotherapy (AHIT) using ozone, which can be used to treat a wide variety of diseases that are resistant to traditional medical therapy.

Today some eight thousand licensed health practitioners (including medical doctors, homeopathic physicians, and naturopaths) in Germany use ozone in their practices, while some fifteen thousand European practitioners use ozone, either alone or as a complement to other therapies. It is estimated that over ten million ozone treatments have been given to over one million patients in Germany alone over the last forty years. While considered experimental by North American scientists, the medical uses of ozone are well known and well established outside the United States.

Research in Medical Ozone

Since the end of World War II, hundreds of laboratory and clinical studies on the medical uses of ozone have been undertaken, primarily in Europe, and the findings have been published in a variety of scientific and medical journals. Most have been published in German, with the exception of those findings first reported at international medical conferences sponsored by the International Ozone Association, which were presented in English. At the present time, the bulk of scientific research in the medical uses of ozone is being conducted in Cuba, Russia, and Germany, where researchers receive the cooperation and support of the government and major universities. Research is going on to a far lesser extent in the United States, France, Italy, Mexico, and Canada.

One recent Canadian study did receive worldwide attention, however. Published in the *Canadian Medical Association Journal*, it showed that ozone kills the human immunodeficiency virus (HIV), the hepatitis and herpes viruses, and other harmful agents in the blood used for transfusion. The article's author added: "The systemic use of ozone in the treatment of AIDS could not only reduce the virus load but also possibly revitalize the immune system."[3]

Some of the most exciting research in ozone therapy is taking place in two unlikely countries: Russia and Cuba. In the former Soviet Union, physicians, chemists, biologists, and other scientists have been working with the support of the Ministry of Public Health at major institutions like the Interregional Cardiovascular Center and the Central Scientific Laboratory at the Medical Institute in Nizhni Novgorod (Gorky), the Sechenov Medical Academy, and the Central Scientific Research Institute of Dermatology and Venerology in Moscow, as well as the Institute of Photobiology in Minsk, Belarus Republic. Ozone therapy has been approved by the Ministry for Public Health. Ozone therapy is fast becoming part of the medical mainstream in Russia, and physicians from around the country are going to Nizhni Novgorod for training.

Medical ozone research has been carried out since 1985 in Cuba under the auspices of the Department of Ozone, a branch of the prestigious National Academy for Scientific Research (CENIC) in Havana. In addition to research in medical ozone, the department is involved in the use of ozone for sanitation and wastewater treatment, as well as the design, construction, and installation of ozone generators. The department also works closely with physicians throughout the country as part of the National Program for Ozone Therapy. Since 1985, over twenty thousand patients have been treated with ozone in medical institutions throughout the country, and many foreigners travel to Cuba for advanced medical therapy, including ozone.

In 1994, the Department of Ozone with its staff of sixty chemists and laboratory technicians moved to a new campus on the outskirts of Havana, the Center for Ozone Research. This modern facility includes two laboratories, two ozone clinics (one for Cubans and one for foreigners), an administration building, and a 180-bed hotel for foreign patients and their families.

It is important to view Cuba's ozone research in the context of the Cuban health-care system. One of the primary goals of the Cuban revolution of 1959 was to provide free and universal health care to all Cuban citizens. Although subjected to a crippling economic blockade by the United States government since 1961, Cuba has nonetheless been able to position itself in the vanguard of medical research in genetic engineering (Cuba's Center for Biotechnology and Genetic Engineering is the first in Latin America), organ transplant technology, the development of an artificial heart, the development of vaccines for hepatitis B and meningococcal meningitis B, use of neural brain implants to treat Parkinson's disease, and use of epidermal growth factor to aid burn victims.[4]

In contrast to his devastating eyewitness account of the disintegration of Castro's Cuba in his book *Castro's Final Hour,* Andrés Oppenheimer had the following to say about the Cuban health-care system:

> In fact, the revolution's greatest success had been in providing a first-class health care system for free. Whatever health needs Cubans had, whether a pregnancy test or a heart-bypass operation, they could have it for the asking. And because health care was the revolution's greatest pride, the state's magnanimity was unlimited: even cosmetic surgery and orthodontic treatments were performed without charge.[5]

Despite severe problems with transportation, agriculture, and economic development, Cuba has consistently maintained one of the highest levels of health care in all of Latin America. The results of much of the Cuban research on ozone therapies are presented to the general lay public for the first time in this book.

Why are the Cubans and Russians so interested in ozone? Citizens of both countries have enjoyed socialized medicine for decades, so private drug manufacturers and private hospitals and clinics have traditionally played a small or nonexistent role in determining the direction of the health-care system. As mentioned before, ozone cannot be patented, it is extremely cheap to produce, and it can be used effectively in a wide range of therapeutical applications. In countries like the United States, where large drug companies are directly or indirectly involved in all medical research and lobby to influence government policy, there is simply no interest in researching the possibilities of ozone therapy. Yet in countries where the profit motive is absent from health care, physicians, chemists, and other researchers traditionally enjoy both government support and government funding for their work.

Properties and Uses of Ozone

We mentioned earlier that ozone is a powerful oxidizer that can kill a wide variety of viruses, bacteria, and other toxins. It also oxidizes phenolics (poisonous compounds of methanol and benzine), pesticides, detergents, chemical manufacturing wastes, and aromatic (smelly) compounds more rapidly and effectively than chlorine, yet without its harmful residues.[6] For this reason, ozone has become the element of choice to disinfect and purify drinking water and wastewater through a wide variety of applications.

Municipal Water Treatment

In an age of increasing pollution of drinking water supplies, ozone is becoming regarded as an inexpensive, safe, and effective purification alternative to chlorine and other substances.

More than a hundred different viruses that are excreted in human feces can be found in contaminated drinking water. Viruses like those associated with hepatitis infect thousands of people a year and survive for a long time in potable water. As a potent virucide, ozone is seen as an effective alternative to chlorine, which (in addition to its undesirable taste and odor) may yield chloroform and other compounds that are potentially carcinogenic.[7] According to *The Encyclopedia of Chemical Technology:*

> Chlorination as it is practiced in potable-water treatment plants cannot adequately remove viruses to an acceptable level. The complete control of viruses by ozone at low dosage levels is well documented.[8]

As a potent oxidizer, ozone kills bacteria by rupturing the cell wall. Among the harmful microorganisms that ozone can oxidize are *Escherichia coli* (E. coli), *Streptococcus fecalis, Mycobacterium tuberculosum, Cryptosporidium parvum, Bacillus megatherium* (spores), and *Endamoeba histolytica. The Encyclopedia of Chemical Technology* reports that

> ozone displays an all-or-nothing effect in terms of destroying bacteria. This effect can be attributed to the high oxidation potential of ozone. Ozone is such a strong germicide that only a few micrograms per liter are required to measure germicidal action.[9]

Today, more than twenty-five hundred municipalities around the world purify their water supplies with ozone, including Los Angeles, Paris, Montreal, Moscow, Kiev, Singapore, Brussels, Florence, Turin, Marseille, Manchester, and Amsterdam.

A 1996 advice column in a weekend supplement to the *Los Angeles Times* spoke highly of using ozone in swimming pools, adding that ozone generators are easy to install and use in residential pools. Speaking of the advantages of ozone over chlorine, the author wrote:

> Activated oxygen, ozone, is one of the best and safest swimming pool and spa purifiers. An ozone purifier can cut chemical usage by 80% and eliminate burning eyes, faded and bleached bathing suits, dry skin, etc.

Many major cities use ozone to purify their drinking water. . . . A very low concentration of ozone gas in water is not harmful to people or pets, but it destroys bacteria, viruses and tiny particles. Within several minutes, ozone converts back to pure oxygen. Ozone gas breaks down bacteria and virus cell-walls in seconds and kills them. Chlorine takes hours to slowly penetrate these cells. Chlorine can react with common compounds in the pool to create cancer-causing chemicals.[10]

Ozone has also been used to purify the water in public swimming pools since 1950. During the Olympic Games in Los Angeles during the summer of 1984, the European teams insisted that the water in the swimming pools be treated with ozone instead of as opposed to chlorine, or they would not participate in the events.

Ozone in Industry

Ozone is used by the bottling industry to disinfect the insides of soda and beer bottles. The ozone later disappears as it decomposes to oxygen. Brewers use ozone to remove any residual bad taste and odor from the water used in beer production. Ozone is also utilized by the pharmaceutical industry as a disinfectant and in the manufacture of electrical components to oxidize surface impurities. Ozone concentrations of one to three parts per million are used to inhibit the growth of molds and bacteria in stored foods like eggs, meat, vegetables, and fruits.[11]

Wastewater Pollution Control

Ozone can break down industrial wastes like phenol and cyanide so that they become biodegradable. It is often used to oxidize mining wastes, wastes from the photographic industry, and harmful compounds like heavy metals, ethanol, and acetic acid.[12]

Ozone is also used to disinfect municipal wastewater and to clean up lakes and streams that have become polluted by sewage and other pollutants. Unlike chlorine, ozone can clean up a lake or stream without killing the resident animal life or leaving potentially harmful chemical residues in the ecosystem.

Air and Odor Treatment

In the United States, over one hundred ozone generators are used by both municipalities and private companies to remove noxious odors from treated sewage. Sewage contains high amounts of foul-smelling chemicals like sulfides, amines, and olefins. Ozone gas does not mask their odors; it oxidates those compounds and renders them odor free.

Ozone is also used to reduce odors in rendering plants, paper mills, compost operations, underground railways, tunnels, and mines. The food industry uses minute amounts of ozone to treat odors in dairies, fish-processing plants, and slaughterhouses.[13]

Ozone in Medicine

The applications of ozone to medical therapy were first documented in European medical journals in the mid-1930s. Since that time, over a thousand articles have been published in medical and scientific journals, mostly in German, Russian, and Spanish.

Used primarily to kill viruses, destroy bacteria, and eliminate fungi, ozone produces important benefits in the human body, including the oxygenation of blood, improved blood circulation, and stimulation of the oxygen-producing facility in human tissues. It is also an important immunoregulator. For these reasons, the range of human health problems that can respond favorably to ozone therapy is quite broad. According to Drs. Siegfried Rilling and Renate Viebahn in their book *The Use of Ozone in Medicine*, physicians have used ozone therapy in the areas of angiology (blood vessels), dermatology (including allergology), gastroenterology, gerontology, intensive care, gynecology, neurology, odontology, oncology, orthopedics, proctology, radiology, rheumatology, surgery (including vascular surgery), and urology.[14] As the Canadian report cited earlier indicated, ozone has been proved to effectively purify human blood supplies.

According to the European-based Medical Society for Ozone (with branches in Germany, Austria, Italy, and Switzerland) and the National Center for Scientific Research in Cuba, physicians are currently treating the following diseases with different forms of ozone therapy:[15]

abscesses
acne
AIDS
allergies (hypersensitivity)
anal fissures
arthritis
arthrosis
asthma
cancerous tumors
cerebral sclerosis
circulatory disturbances
cirrhosis of the liver
climacterium (menopause)
constipation
corneal ulcers
cystitis
decubitus ulcers (bedsores)
diarrhea
fistulae
fungal diseases
furunculosis
gangrene
gastro-duodenal ulcers
gastro-intestinal disorders
giardiasis

glaucoma
hepatitis
herpes (simplex and zoster)
hypercholesterolemia
mucous colitis
mycosis
nerve-related disorders
    osteomyelitis
Parkinson's disease
polyarthritis
Raynaud's disease
retinitis pigmentosa
rheumatoid arthritis
scars (after radiation)
senile dementia
sepsis control
sinusitis
spondylitis
stomatitis
Sudeck's disease
thrombophlebitis
ulcus cruris (open leg sores)
vulvovaginitis
wound-healing disturbances

Ozone in the Dentist's Office

Since one of the pioneers in ozone therapy was a dentist, it is important to mention that ozone has a place in dental practice. According to the German dentist Fritz Kramer, ozone in the form of ozonated water can be effective in the following ways:

- as a powerful disinfectant
- in its ability to control bleeding
- in its ability to cleanse wounds in bones and soft tissue
- to speed healing by improving the local supply of oxygen to the wound area
- to improve the metabolic processes related to healing by increasing temperature in the area of the wound

Dr. Kramer points out that ozonated water can be used in several different applications:

- as a mouth rinse (especially in cases of gingivitis, paradentosis, thrush, or stomatitis)
- as a spray to cleanse the affected area and to disinfect oral mucosa and cavities and in general dental surgery
- as an ozone–water jet to clean cavities of teeth being capped or receiving root canal therapy[16]

How Is Ozone Therapy Applied?

Over the past sixty years, more than a dozen methods have been developed in the application of ozone in medical therapy. In most cases, tiny amounts of ozone are added to pure oxygen (usually 0.05 parts of ozone to 99.95 parts of oxygen for internal use and 5 parts of ozone to 95 parts of oxygen for external applications). This is usually expressed in terms of micrograms of ozone per milliliter of oxygen ($\mu g/ml$). For example, if a physician were to require 1200 μg of ozone, he or she would select a concentration of 12 $\mu g/ml$ and use a volume of 100 ml of oxygen. The exact amount is determined on a case-by-case basis, as physicians have found that not enough ozone can be ineffective, while too much can be immunosuppressive. At the present time, eight simple methods and one highly complex method of ozone therapy are used in medical practice.

Direct Intra-arterial Application

In this method, used primarily for arterial circulatory disorders, an ozone–oxygen mixture is slowly injected into an artery or vein with a hypodermic syringe. According to Gerard V. Sunnen, M.D., "Due to accidents produced by too rapid introduction of the gas mixture into the circulation, this technique is now rarely used."[17]

Rectal Insufflation

In rectal insufflation, first pioneered by Payr and Aubourg in the 1930s, a mixture of ozone and oxygen is introduced through the rectum and absorbed into the body through the intestine. Typically, approximately 100–800 ml of oxygen and ozone (for an average adult of normal body weight) is insufflated into the rectum, a process that takes between ninety seconds and two minutes. The oxygen–ozone is then retained in the intestine for ten to twenty minutes.

Used for a wide variety of health problems, this method is considered one of the safest. In a typical treatment for ulcerative colitis, 75 µg of ozone per milliliter of oxygen are used (treatment begins with 50 ml of oxygen, which can be increased slowly to 500 ml per treatment).[18] While administered under medical supervision in Germany, Russia, and Cuba, this method is used by a growing number of people in the United States for self-treatment of cancer, HIV-related problems, and other diseases.

Dr. Horst Kief believes that rectal insufflation is a valuable method of ozone–oxygen delivery due to several unique properties of the large intestine, especially its enormous surface of resorption.

1. The intestinum of adults is approx. 12 meters long and due to the multitude of intestinal villi and crypts features a surface of 10 square meters.

2. The lymphatic system of the intestinum, i.e., Peyer's patches, occupy more space within the human organism than is used by the spleen and the thymus together.

3. The circulatory system of the intestinum is directly connected to the liver through the portal vein, where most of the biochemical, immunological and metabolic processes take place.

4. "Death lives in the intestines"—this popular saying presumably is derived from the deeply rooted archaic knowledge that the intestinal flora—the pathological flora in particular—may trigger a number of diseases, which most frequently is misjudged or rather underestimated by traditional medicine.

Considering the anatomic, immunological, biochemical and microbiological particularities of the intestinum, the use of Medical Ozone should reasonably be expected to provide decisive therapeutical consequences in rectal application, and to yield successful clinical results.

He adds that the use of medical ozone in rectal application:

1. should provide for measurable resorption to be obtained upon insufflation of sufficient volumes.

2. should provide for a substantial immunological effect to be obtained due to direct contamination of the largest lymphatic system of the human organism.

3. should yield improvements relating to all oxidative processes taking place in the liver due to the increased flood of reactive oxygen metabolites supplied to this organ.

4. should provide for the microbiological milieu to be improved in cases of pathological changes of the intestinal flora due to old age and wrongful eating habits within our society.[19]

Intramuscular Injection

In intramuscular injection, a small amount of an ozone and oxygen mixture (up to 10 ml) is injected into the patient (usually in the buttocks) as a normal injection would be. This method is commonly used to treat allergies and inflammatory diseases. Intramuscular injections are sometimes used as an adjunct to cancer therapies in Europe.

Major and Minor Autohemotherapy

Used since the 1960s, *minor autohemotherapy* involves removing a small amount (usually 10 ml) of the patient's blood from a vein with a hypodermic syringe, treating it with ozone and oxygen, and giving it back to the patient via intramuscular injection. Thus the blood and ozone become a type of autovaccine that is derived from the patient's own cells and can be very specific and effective in treating the patient's health problem.

Major autohemotherapy typically calls for the removal of up to 250 ml of the patient's blood. Ozone and oxygen are bubbled into the blood for several minutes, and then the ozonated blood is reintroduced into the vein in the form of an IV drip.

These methods have been used successfully to treat a wide variety of health problems, including herpes, arthritis, cancer, heart disease, and HIV infection. It is probably the most commonly used type of ozone therapy today. Figure 2.3 shows the four steps used to deliver ozone through major autohemotherapy.

Ozonated Water

This method calls for ozone gas to be bubbled through water, and then the water is used externally to bathe wounds, burns, and slow-healing skin infections. It is also used as a disinfectant by dentists who perform dental surgery. In Russia, physicians use ozonated water to irrigate body cavities during surgery. In both Russia and Cuba, ozonated water is used to treat a wide variety of intestinal and gynecological problems, including ulcerative colitis, duodenal ulcers, gastritis, diarrhea, and vulvovaginitis.[20] Ozonated water can also be used for colonics or enemas.

Intra-articular Injection

In this method, ozone gas is bubbled through water, and then the mixture is injected directly between the joints. It is used primarily by physicians in Germany, Russia, and Cuba to treat arthritis, rheumatism, and other joint diseases.

Intravenous Injection

This controversial method involves injecting a mixture of oxygen and ozone directly into a vein. Although a number of physicians in the United States and Canada found this method to be both safe and more effective than major autohemotherapy, European and Cuban doctors consider it dangerous and without clinical advantages over other ozone delivery methods.

In a monograph on ozone therapy, Dr. Velio Bocci, a world leader in research in medical ozone at the Institute of General Physiology at

Figure 2.3. Major autohemotherapy, Cira García Hospital, Havana. (Photos by Nathaniel Altman.)
  1. One half pint of blood is removed from the patient.
  2. Ozone is taken from medical ozone generator with a syringe.
  3. The ozone is injected into the blood.
  4. The ozonated blood is then slowly reinfused into the patient.

the University of Siena in Italy, cautioned: "Use of the intravenous administration route is extremely dangerous because even if the gaseous mixture of oxygen-ozone is administered very slowly with a pump, it frequently procures lung embolization and serious side effects, particularly when daily dosing is up to 120 ml." He also points out that in a 1983 German survey on the safety of ozone applications, the only adverse side effects among patients surveyed were attributed to IV injection. Administering ozone through this method is presently outlawed in Germany.[21]

Steam Cabinet Method

This noninvasive method is becoming increasingly popular among patients and practitioners. The patient enters a steam cabinet and, in addition to steam, a mixture of oxygen and ozone is pumped into the cabinet through a tube connected to an ozone generator. It is believed that the body absorbs the ozone through the skin, which eventually finds its way into the bloodstream. This method is described in detail in chapter 8.

Ear Insufflation

Applying ozone and oxygen through the ear is a recent development in ozone therapy. This unconventional method is based on the idea that ozone is absorbed by the body through the tiny capillaries in the ear canal.

Used only in a well-ventilated room (and preferably with a fan placed behind the patient to prevent possible inhalation of ozone), the ozone generator is connected to a tube with a plastic catheter. The generator is turned on and the catheter is placed gently but firmly into the ear, allowing no gas to escape. Ozone and oxygen will enter the ear for one or two minutes. When the patient is able to smell the ozone, it is supposed to indicate that the body has absorbed the ozone it needs. Typically, sick patients undergo three treatments a week. Although this method has not been clinically studied, there is anecdotal evidence that it is both safe and effective in maintaining health and treating disease.

Ozone Bagging

This noninvasive method uses a specially made airtight plastic bag that is placed around the area to be treated. An ozone–oxygen mixture is pumped into the bag, and the mixture is absorbed into the body through the skin. Ozone bagging is primarily recommended for treating leg ulcers, gangrene, fungal infections, burns, and slow-healing wounds.

Ozone in a "sauna bag" (which leaves the head uncovered) is now being used to treat more generalized health problems, such as HIV infection. Typically, the patient takes a warm shower and gets into the bag. Pure oxygen mixed with small amounts of ozone is then pumped into the bag for twenty to thirty minutes, making contact with all skin surfaces. The skin absorbs the ozone. According to Dr. Sunnen, "Surprisingly, the mixture is able to penetrate far enough into the capillary networks to raise blood oxygen pressure. Presumably then, ozone is able to exert its biochemical influence."[22]

Ozonated Oil

Ozonated oil has been used to treat skin problems for over a century. Although not yet widely available in pharmacies, it became quite popular in Europe during the 1950s and is marketed by mail through a number of ozone suppliers in the United States and Canada (see resources section). Ozone gas is added to olive oil and applied as a balm or salve for long-term, low-dose exposure. Other bases (such as sunflower oil) for salves and creams have been developed in Cuba, where their effects have been extensively documented in hospitals and clinics.

Ozonized oil has been found to be useful in treating a wide variety of skin problems, including dermatitis, bacterial infections of the skin (including staphylococcal diseases such as cellulitis, impetigo, ecthyma, and scalded skin syndrome), fungal infections (including infections of the nail bed and athlete's foot), fistulae, leg ulcers, bedsores, gingivitis, herpes simplex, hemorrhoids, vulvovaginitis, bee stings and insect bites, acne, furuncles and carbuncles, infections of the sweat glands (hidradenitis suppurativa), and yeast infections of the skin including candidiasis (caused by Candida albicans). It is also useful in the postsurgical treatment of wounds, and Cuban physicians are using capsules filled with ozonated oil to treat gastro-duodenal ulcers, gastritis, giardiasis, and peptic ulcers.

Inhalation of Ozone

The lungs are the organs most sensitive to ozone. Physicians who use medical ozone warn that inhaling ozone into the lungs can bring about alterations in the density of the lung tissue, damage delicate lung membranes, irritate the epithelium (the surface layer of mucous membrane) in the trachea and bronchi, and lead to emphysema. They also caution users that no ozone should escape into the room in which it is being used; properly designed medical ozone generators are becoming available for use in avoiding the accidental escape of ozone gas. Dr. Stephen A. Levine, the co-author of *Antioxidant Adaptation*, cautions people against using commercial air purifiers that generate small amounts of ozone to clean the air, since ozone should not be inhaled.

This having been said, it is important to point out that in Russia, tiny amounts of ozone are being added to oxygen for short-term therapeutic inhalation in certain cases. This has been done with patients suffering from carbon monoxide poisoning, and doctors have been impressed with the results. No adverse effects were observed.[23] However, by bubbling ozone and oxygen into olive oil, a different gas ($C_{10}H_{18}O_3$) that can be safely inhaled through the nostrils is produced. Alternative healers have found that breathing this gas through a mask is both safe and effective for treating asthma and other respiratory diseases.

Autohomologous Immunotherapy (AHIT)

This method of ozone therapy was developed by the German physician Horst Kief in the early 1980s. It is a patented method of therapy, a new form of autohemotherapy, currently used by over 120 physicians in Europe. AHIT is not approved for use in the United States.

The patient's own blood and urine are taken to a laboratory and are broken down into their different cellular and fluid parts, known as *fractions*. Each fraction undergoes more than a dozen special biochemical and processing steps, including ozonization. These different fractions are then recombined according to the individual's diagnosis and administered as drops, injections, or inhalation fluids over a period of several months.

AHIT has been found to have a strong influence on the immune system. It causes a change in the immunological cell systems that aid in stimulating the body's natural defense mechanisms. Unlike antibiotics and other medications, AHIT has produced no adverse side effects in literally thousands of applications. AHIT has been clinically shown to have a potent effect on a wide range of diseases, like cancer, eczema, bronchial asthma, allergies, rheumatic joint diseases, chronic infections, and premature aging. It also holds promise for the treatment of other diseases like hepatitis, HIV-related problems, cirrhosis, and ulcerative colitis.[24]

Different therapies require specific concentrations of ozone. Some generators, like the German and Cuban machines illustrated earlier in this chapter, are capable of generating ozone for all therapeutic applications, while others (especially inexpensive models designed primarily for tap water treatment in the home) do not. This is why it is important to verify a generator's capability before purchase. Figure 2.4 illustrates the typical concentrations of ozone required for different therapeutic applications.

In part II, we will examine how these different forms of ozone therapy have been used successfully to treat a wide range of specific health problems, both alone and as an adjunct to other forms of medical treatment.

Different applications of ozone

Figure 2.4. Different applications of ozone.
(Graphic reproduced courtesy of Ozone Services.)

3

HYDROGEN PEROXIDE

Hydrogen peroxide is a clear, colorless liquid that easily mixes with water. It is a compound made up of two hydrogen atoms and two oxygen atoms and is known chemically as H_2O_2. Hydrogen Peroxide is created in the atmosphere when ultraviolet light strikes oxygen in the presence of moisture. Ozone (O_3) is free oxygen (O_2) plus an extra atom of oxygen. When it comes into contact with water, this extra atom of oxygen splits off very easily. Water (H_2O) combines with the extra atom of oxygen and becomes hydrogen peroxide (H_2O_2).

We can call hydrogen peroxide a close relative of ozone. Aside from being known as a powerful oxygenator and oxidizer, a special quality of hydrogen peroxide is its ability to readily decompose into water and oxygen. Like ozone, hydrogen peroxide reacts easily with other substances and is able to kill bacteria, fungi, parasites, viruses, and some types of tumor cells.

Hydrogen peroxide occurs naturally within the Earth's biosphere; traces of it are found in rain and snow. It has also been found in many of the healing springs of the world, including Fatima in Portugal, Lourdes in France, and the Shrine of St. Anne in Quebec. Hydrogen peroxide is an important component of plant life, and small amounts are found in many vegetables and fruits, including fresh cabbage, tomatoes, asparagus, green peppers, watercress, oranges, apples, and watermelons.[1]

Hydrogen peroxide is also found in the animal kingdom and is involved in many of our body's natural processes. As an oxygenator, it is able to deliver small quantities of oxygen to the blood and other vital systems throughout the body. Hydrogen peroxide does not oxygenate the body merely by producing modest amounts of oxygen, however; it has an extraordinary capacity to stimulate oxidative enzymes, which have the ability to change the chemical component of other substances (like viruses and bacteria) without being changed themselves. Rather than providing more oxygen to the cells, the presence of hydrogen peroxide *enhances* natural cellular oxidative processes, which increases the body's ability to use what oxygen is available. According to Charles H. Farr, M.D., Ph.D., one of the world's leading authorities on the chemical properties and therapeutic applications of hydrogen peroxide:

> It functions to aid [cell] membrane transport, acts as a hormonal messenger, regulates thermogenesis (heat production), stimulates and regulates immune functions, regulates energy production [similar to insulin] and has many other important metabolic functions. It is purposely used by the body to produce Hydroxyl radicals to kill bacteria, virus, fungi, yeast and a number of parasites. This natural killing or protective system has nothing to do with increasing the amount of available oxygen.[2]

Hydrogen peroxide must be present for our immune system to function properly. The cells in the body that fight infection (the class of white blood cells known as granulocytes) produce hydrogen peroxide as a first line of defense against harmful parasites, bacteria, viruses, and fungi. Hydrogen peroxide is also needed for the metabolism of protein, carbohydrates, fats, vitamins, and minerals. It is a by-product of cell metabolism (that is actively broken down by peroxidase), a hormonal regulator, and a necessary part of the body's production of estrogen, progesterone, and thyroxin. If that weren't enough, hydrogen peroxide is involved in the regulation of blood sugar and the production of energy in body cells.[3]

History and Characteristics

Hydrogen peroxide was discovered in 1818 by the French chemist Louis-Jacques Thenard, who named it *eau oxygenée*, or "oxygenated water." It has been used commercially since the mid-1800s as a nonpolluting bleaching agent, oxidizing agent, and disinfectant.

Although it is found in nature, small quantities of hydrogen peroxide can be made in the laboratory by reacting barium peroxide with cold diluted sulfuric acid. Larger amounts are produced by electrolyzing chilled concentrated sulfuric acid. This process causes a series of chemical reactions to occur and to create a substance called peroxy-disulfuric acid. When the solution is warmed to room temperature, it becomes hydrogen peroxide.[4]

Hydrogen peroxide is found in a variety of different grades:

- *3 percent grade hydrogen peroxide* is the type we find in pharmacies and grocery stores. Made primarily of 50 percent "super D peroxide" and diluted, it contains a variety of stabilizers like phenol, acetanilide, and sodium stancite. It is used mostly to disinfect wounds and treat skin rashes, and as an effective, inexpensive (although unpleasant tasting to some) mouthwash. This grade of hydrogen peroxide is also used around the house to freshen the bathroom and to wash fresh fruits and vegetables. While safe for those applications, 3 percent grade H_2O_2 should not be ingested.

- *6 percent grade hydrogen peroxide* contains an activator that makes it an effective bleaching agent. It is used primarily by hairdressers, surfers, and teenagers for coloring their hair.

- Like other grades of hydrogen peroxide, *30 percent reagent grade* looks like harmless water. However, it is a highly concentrated chemical compound that is very corrosive. Strict precautions must be taken by those who plan to use it. When it makes contact with skin, burns can result. Breathing the vapor or ingesting it full strength can be hazardous and even fatal. Yet when used properly, reagent-grade hydrogen peroxide is safe. Because it is relatively free of heavy metals and other trace elements, it is used primarily in medical research. It is also highly recommended for use (in diluted form) in bio-oxidative therapy. Reagent-grade hydrogen peroxide can be found in chemical supply stores.

- *35 percent food-grade hydrogen peroxide* has traditionally been used by the food industry as a nontoxic disinfectant. Added to water, it is sprayed on cheese, eggs, vegetables, fruits, and whey products to keep them free of unwanted bacteria. It is used to disinfect metal and foil-lined food containers. Food-grade hydrogen peroxide is also used in the dairy industry as a disinfectant and bactericide. While considered less desirable than reagent grade for use in bio-oxidative therapy, food-grade hydrogen peroxide is easily obtainable in any large natural-food store.

- *90 percent hydrogen peroxide* is used by the military and in space exploration as a propulsion source for rocket fuel. A highly unstable compound that can explode unless handled very carefully, it is *not* recommended for use in bio-oxidative therapy.

Major Uses

Like ozone, hydrogen peroxide is used in a variety of ways:

Bleaching

One of the major industrial uses of hydrogen peroxide is in the bleaching of cotton textiles, while it is used to a lesser extent to bleach wool, silk, and certain vegetable fibers. It is also used to bleach chemical pulps, groundwood, and linoleum and to improve the color of certain waxes and oils. Hydrogen peroxide is used to de-ink waste paper in the recycling process. These industries like using hydrogen peroxide because it is environmentally friendly. When hydrogen peroxide decomposes, it yields only water and oxygen.

Pollution Control

Hydrogen peroxide also is a powerful oxidizer, bactericide, and virucide. When added to industrial and residential sewage and wastewaters, it kills harmful pathogens, making those effluents safe for the environment. Hydrogen peroxide removes toxic and foul-smelling pollutants from industrial gas streams and can limit chlorine concentration in water supplies.

Chemicals, Pharmaceuticals, and Mining

Hydrogen peroxide is utilized by the chemical industry in the production of a wide variety of organic and inorganic chemicals, as well as in the manufacture of household bleaches. It is an ingredient in contact lens cleaners, eye drops, aloe vera extracts, and mouthwashes. Hydrogen peroxide is also an oxidizing agent in the mining industry.

Propellant

High-grade (90 percent) hydrogen peroxide is used as a rocket fuel by different branches of the armed forces and the National Aeronautics and Space Administration (NASA).

Agriculture

As an inexpensive way for farmers to purify drinking water, one pint of 35 percent food-grade hydrogen peroxide is added to one thousand gallons of drinking water for farm animals. In addition to serving as a catalyst for promoting oxygenation of the blood and killing harmful viruses and bacteria, hydrogen peroxide added to drinking water helps eliminate worms and other parasites from the intestine. When given to dairy cows, it can increase both the production of milk and its butterfat content.

One farmer related his experience with hydrogen peroxide:

In 1990, I was administering 35% H_2O_2 orally to bovines (a dairy herd), at 30 ppm, added to their drinking water. All the water on the farm was treated, so it was also in all cleanup water, etc. That's a low dose. Somebody must know how to convert it to percentage or whatever they want. I know how, but I'm not big on technical points. The cows became extremely healthy. Bacteria counts dropped and butterfat went up. Those two criteria convert immediately to money for the farmer. He is paid more for his milk the very next pickup. So, I started taking it myself.[5]

Food-grade hydrogen peroxide is used to rinse milk cans and bulk tanks to destroy bacteria and other pathogens. It is also diluted with water and used as a spray to clean barn walls and floors. Hydrogen peroxide mixtures are used to clean wounds and wash the udders of cows, which results in a lower bacteria content in their milk.

Because oxygen is essential for plant life as well as animal life, hydrogen peroxide is being used in various ways to increase the growth rate and productivity of plants. Farmgard Products of Minnesota reports that nonbearing fruit trees grew fruit when given water containing hydrogen peroxide and nonproductive rice paddies in Japan bore crops after being irrigated with water mixed with hydrogen peroxide. Hydrogen peroxide is also used by some farmers to make an effective non-polluting insecticide in the field as well as a spray for home and garden plants.[6]

Hydrogen Peroxide in Medicine

The first medical use of hydrogen peroxide was reported by I. N. Love, M.D., a consulting physician at the City Hospital in St. Louis, in the March 3, 1888, issue of the *Journal of the American Medical Association* under the title "Peroxide of Hydrogen as a Remedial Agent." The article, based on a talk given to the St. Louis Medical Society the previous month, related Dr. Love's success in treating patients with a variety of diseases, including scarlet fever, diphtheria, nasal catarrh, acute coryza (head catarrh), whooping cough, asthma, hay fever, and tonsillitis. In these cases, treatment primarily involved administering a diluted solution of hydrogen peroxide into the nostrils with a syringe. Dr. Love commented: "From its very nature this agent should be a powerful antiseptic and a destroyer of microbes; anything which accomplishes oxidation as rapidly, if it can be applied safely, must be an excellent application to purulent surfaces for its cleansing effect." The author also mentioned its use (unsuccessfully) in treating diabetes and addresses possible clinical applications in treating some forms of atonic dyspepsia and gonorrhea. Dr. Love observed: "The beneficial effect of the application was apparent, all the distressing symptoms were much abated, and within three or four days they had passed away. . . ." Dr. Love also documented the use of hydrogen peroxide in treating uterine cancer as a "cleanser, deodorizer and stimulator of healing."[7]

Later that year at the Annual Meeting of the Medical Society of Georgia, P. R. Cortelyou, M.D., reported his clinical experience with hydrogen peroxide in treating disorders of the throat and nose. Dr. Cortelyou diluted hydrogen peroxide and used the fluid as a fine spray for treating people with chronic pharyngitis, rhinitis, cough, sore throat tonsillitis, and diphtheria. In some cases, Dr. Cortelyou used hydrogen peroxide in combination with other medicines of the time, including "muriate of cocaine," and a solution made with iodine, potash, and glycerine. After treating a woman suffering from severe cough and high fever with this combination for four weeks, the doctor reported: "The throat was feeling so much better that the treatment was only given twice a week, and patient has kept in good condition all winter."[8]

The first known use of intravenous hydrogen peroxide was reported by the British physician T. H. Oliver in 1920. In India the previous year he had treated twenty-five patients who were critically ill with influenzal pneumonia by injecting hydrogen peroxide directly into their veins.

Compared to a typical death rate of over 80 percent for this disease, Oliver's patients had a mortality rate of only 48 percent.[9] Although this method of hydrogen peroxide delivery can cause gas embolism, a condition that can obstruct blood vessels and lead to a stroke, apparently that did not occur in any of the patients treated.

In the United States, studies with hydrogen peroxide were conducted by the noted chemist and physician William Frederick Koch in the 1920s with cancer patients. Dr. Koch used a substance he called glyoxylide, which is believed to be the same oxygen found in hydrogen peroxide. Rather than using intravenous administration like Oliver, he preferred giving the substance intramuscularly.

While his treatments were successful, Dr. Koch was later sued by the United States Food and Drug Administration. Although acquitted, he decided to leave the United States and continue his research in Brazil. He died there in 1967.[10]

In the early 1960s, major studies in the medical uses of hydrogen peroxide were conducted at the Baylor University Medical Center in Texas. In an early study involving cancer, researchers found that cells containing a high amount of oxygen responded more favorably to radiation therapy than ordinary cells. Before that study, hyperbaric oxygen was often used by physicians to oxygenate the cells; in a rather cumbersome and expensive method using a specially built oxygen chamber, oxygen was delivered under pressure greater than normal atmospheric pressure. However, the doctors at Baylor found that small amounts of hydrogen peroxide injected into a vein could achieve the same effect as hyperbaric oxygen at a much lower cost and with fewer adverse side effects.

The Baylor researchers also discovered that hydrogen peroxide has an energizing effect on the heart muscle that could be of great benefit to patients suffering heart attacks. Myocardial ischemia, or lack of oxygen to the heart muscle, was relieved with hydrogen peroxide.[11] Writing in the journal *Circulation*, Dr. H. C. Urschel Jr., reported that ventricular fibrillation—a life-threatening condition involving extremely rapid, incomplete contractions of the ventricle area of the heart—was completely relieved through the intravenous administration of hydrogen peroxide.[12]

The researchers at Baylor also studied the effect of intravenous hydrogen peroxide on the accumulation of plaque in the arteries. They found not only that hydrogen peroxide removed plaque buildup efficiently but also that its effects were long term.[13] While those findings offered hope to individuals destined for expensive, dangerous, and often ineffective heart bypass operations, the Baylor studies were largely ignored by the medical establishment. They are presented in more detail in part II of this book.

Perhaps the most important medical research in hydrogen peroxide therapy today can be credited to Charles H. Farr of Oklahoma, who holds doctoral degrees in both pharmacology and medicine. Dr. Farr was among the first to suggest the clinical benefits of treating illnesses with diluted solutions of hydrogen peroxide injected intravenously, and he has conducted more clinical research in the fields of chelation therapy and hydrogen peroxide therapy than anyone else. In addition to having written over thirty-five scientific and medical articles and books, he is the founder of the International Oxidative Medicine Association (IOMA).

Like that of many pioneers who have researched the value of the medical applications of ozone, Dr. Farr's work in hydrogen peroxide has been largely ignored by the scientific and medical establishments in the United States and Canada. However, it has been carefully evaluated by eminent scientists abroad. In recognition of his accomplishments in the field of hydrogen peroxide therapy and research in biological oxidation, Dr. Farr was nominated to receive the 1993 Nobel Prize for Medicine.

How Does It Work?

We mentioned before that hydrogen peroxide is both an effective oxygenator and a powerful oxidizer. Numerous physiological effects of hydrogen peroxide have been described in medical and scientific literature for over sixty years.

On the Lungs

Hydrogen peroxide helps stimulate the process of oxygenation in the lungs by increasing blood flow, so that blood has more contact with air; it also helps red blood cells and hemoglobin carry oxygen to the cells of the lungs. This helps remove foreign material, including dead and damaged tissue, from the alveoli, the tiny air sacs in the lungs where oxygen is taken into the bloodstream.

On Metabolism

A number of hormonal effects are regulated by the actions of hydrogen peroxide, including the production of progesterone and thyroxine as well as the inhibition of bioamines, dopamine, noradrenalin, and serotonin. Hydrogen peroxide also stimulates (either directly or indirectly) certain oxidative enzyme systems. Enzymes are complex proteins that are able to bring about chemical changes in other substances; digestive enzymes, for example, are able to break down foods into simpler compounds that the body can use for nourishment.

On the Heart and Circulatory System

Hydrogen peroxide can dilate (expand) blood vessels in the heart, the extremities, the brain, and the lungs. It is also able to decrease heart rate, increase stroke volume (the amount of blood pumped by the left ventricle of the heart at each beat), and decrease vascular resistance (which makes it easier for blood to move through the blood vessels). As a result, it can increase total cardiac output.

Sugar (Glucose) Utilization

Hydrogen peroxide is said to mimic the effects of insulin and has been used successfully to stabilize cases of diabetes mellitus type II.

Immune Response

We mentioned before that granulocytes are a type of white blood cell that the body uses to fight infections. When the body is infused with hydrogen peroxide, the number of granulocytes in the body first goes down and then increases beyond the original number.

Intravenous treatment with hydrogen peroxide has also been found to stimulate the formation of monocytes, a type of white blood cell that scavenges, hunts, and kills bacteria; stimulates T-helper cells (white blood cells that orchestrate the immune response and signal other cells in the immune system to perform their special functions); and helps increase the production of gamma interferon, a protein found when cells are exposed to viruses as well as other cytokines (cellular messengers) that promote healing. Noninfected cells that are exposed to interferon become protected against viral infection.[14]

What Diseases Can Hydrogen Peroxide Treat?

Low-grade (3 percent) hydrogen peroxide is well known to most of us. When we apply it externally to an open wound, it bubbles, which is the oxygen coming out of solution. However, few people know about the wide range of therapeutic possibilities of 30 percent reagent-grade or 35 percent food-grade hydrogen peroxide when diluted and taken internally as bio-oxidative therapy.

Like ozone, hydrogen peroxide can treat a broad spectrum of diseases because it kills bacteria, fungi, parasites, and viruses. It can also destroy certain tumor cells. According to Dr. Farr, the following diseases have been clinically treated with intravenous hydrogen peroxide with varying degrees of success:

acute and chronic viral infections

allergies[15]

Alzheimer's disease

angina

asthma

cardiac arrhythmias (irregular heartbeat)

cardioconversion (heart stoppage)

cardiovascular disease (heart disease)

cerebral vascular disease (stroke and memory loss)

chronic obstructive pulmonary disease

chronic pain syndromes (from various causes)

chronic recurrent Epstein–Barr infection

chronic unresponsive bacterial infections

cluster headaches

diabetes mellitus type II

emphysema

herpes simplex (fever blister)

herpes zoster (shingles)

HIV-related infections

influenza

metastatic carcinoma (cancer)

migraine headaches

multiple sclerosis

parasitic infections

Parkinson's disease
peripheral vascular disease (poor circulation)
rheumatoid arthritis
systemic chronic candidiasis (yeast infections)
temporal arteritis (inflammation of the temporal artery)
vascular headaches

In part II, we examine the impact of hydrogen peroxide on many of these health problems in greater detail.

Researchers are currently working on developing treatment protocols for many other diseases, including Legionnaires' disease, Erlich's carcinoma, AIDS-related pneumonia caused by *pneumocystis carinii,* and infections caused by *Candida albicans, Salmonella typhi, Toxoplasma gondii,* cytomegalovirus, and HIV.

How Is Hydrogen Peroxide Administered?

Hydrogen peroxide can be introduced into the body in a number of different ways.

Intravenous Infusion

An intravenous infusion is prepared by diluting 30 percent reagent hydrogen peroxide with an equal amount of sterile distilled water to make a 15 percent "stock solution." This is then passed through a Millipore 0.22-μm medium-flow filter both to sterilize the solution and to remove any particulate matter from it. The stock solution is refrigerated in 100-ml sterile containers until needed.

At the time of application, physicians use 5 percent dextrose in water, or normal saline solution as the carrier. Adding 0.4 ml of the stock solution to 200 ml of dextrose in water results in a 0.03 percent concentration, which is the recommended strength for most intravenous infusions. Because of the tremendous oxidizing power of hydrogen peroxide, Dr. Farr cautions that "vitamins, minerals, peptides, enzymes, amino acids, heparin, EDTA or other injectable materials should never be mixed with the H_2O_2 solution."[16] The mixture is then slowly infused into a vein over a period of one to three hours, depending on the patient's situation. According to the International Oxidative Medicine Association:

Treatments are usually given about once a week in chronic illness but can be given daily in patients with acute illness such as pneumonia or flu. Physicians may recommend 1 to 20 treatments, depending on the condition of the patient and the illness being treated.[17]

Follow-up treatments are sometimes necessary. Although adverse side effects are rare (some people experience irritation in the vein or slight temporary pressure in the chest), the patient is often monitored by a doctor or nurse during and shortly after the infusion.

Because the hydrogen peroxide solution is administered in exact amounts, this is the method most preferred by physicians. It is also considered the most efficient way to introduce hydrogen peroxide into the body.

Oral Ingestion

The oral method calls for drops of 35 percent hydrogen peroxide to be added to a glass of water and ingested two to three times daily. One of the more prominent advocates of this method is the renowned heart surgeon, Dr. Christiaan Barnard. In a letter dated March 10, 1986, he wrote: "It is true that I have found relief from the arthritis and I attribute it to taking hydrogen peroxide orally several times a day."[18]

Kurt W. Donsbach, D.C., the noted holistic practitioner and writer, uses hydrogen peroxide and other natural substances to treat patients with cancer, heart disease, and other illnesses at his Hospital Santa Monica in Mexico. Although Dr. Donsbach prefers the intravenous method at the hospital (and estimates that he and his staff have administered over 120,000 hydrogen peroxide infusions without significant side effects), he recommends oral administration for outpatient use in a product he created known as Superoxy Plus, made from aloe vera saturated with magnesium peroxide. Each ounce is said to be equivalent to twenty drops by hydrogen peroxide.[19]

The well-known lay researcher Conrad LeBeau suggests that adults take ten drops of food-grade hydrogen peroxide in an eight-ounce glass of distilled water two or three times a day on an empty stomach. Donsbach recommends that the mixture be taken on an empty stomach thirty minutes before eating or three hours after eating.[20]

Some people find the taste of hydrogen peroxide unpleasant. To help disguise the taste, several drops of olive oil can be added to the water.

One can also begin taking one drop of hydrogen peroxide in a glass of water on the first day and add a drop per glass each day until ten drops per day are achieved. Dr. Donsbach cautions against taking hydrogen peroxide with juice, milk, or other flavorings, because it will "create oxidation, robbing the oxygen, which is what you are trying to get into the blood stream,"[21] while Dr. Farr notes that "almost without exception, hydrogen peroxide, added to anything besides oil and/or water, will cause dismutation and destruction of the hydrogen peroxide."[22]

Physicians also caution against adding hydrogen peroxide to water containing iron, because the combination of hydrogen peroxide and iron produces a high number of free radicals and can promote stomach upset, possibly leading to cancer over the long term. If one's water contains iron, distilled water is recommended instead. It is also suggested that iron supplements not be taken within an hour of ingesting hydrogen peroxide.

Among the physicians who advocate the use of hydrogen peroxide, not all are in favor of using it orally. One of those critics is Dr. Farr. In addition to the presence of iron in the stomach, he believes that combinations of fatty acids may reduce hydrogen peroxide to a number of free radicals, thus causing negative effects upon the gastric and duodenal mucosa, the delicate membrane lining the stomach and the first part of the small intestine. This may lead to an increase of glandular stomach erosion, an abnormal increase in the number of cells in the duodenum, and the possible formation of cancerous and noncancerous tumors in the stomach and duodenum.[23]

Dr. Farr's views are supported by Hugo Vietz, M.D., a Pennsylvania practitioner who has also had extensive experience using hydrogen peroxide therapeutically. In an article published in *East West* magazine, he strongly discouraged the oral self-administration of hydrogen peroxide:

> You're putting a fairly caustic substance into the intestinal tract, which, from the mouth to the rectum, is lined with a highly sensitive, delicate, multi-purpose mucous membrane. This membrane has some extremely important functions to perform. Introduce a caustic substance like hydrogen peroxide even in the dilute concentrations that they are using, and it scares me. A lot of people who are doing it are going to get away with it. But there are going to be some who will wind up with damaged intestinal tracts. If you cause permanent damage to an organ like this, I think you're in for real trouble.[24]

This subject of oral self-administration of hydrogen peroxide is a controversial one, since many long-term users of oral hydrogen peroxide have not become sick and clinical studies are lacking. Until such studies are done, many feel that the use of oral hydrogen peroxide should be avoided in favor of less risky applications.

In Bathing

A much safer (and less controversial) method involves adding one pint of 35 percent food-grade hydrogen peroxide to a bathtub of warm water and soaking in the water for a minimum of twenty minutes. The hydrogen peroxide is absorbed by the skin. People have reported relief from stiff joints, rashes, psoriasis, and fungal infections by using this method one to three times a week. There is little clinical evidence attesting to the effectiveness of this method in treating serious diseases, but there is much anecdotal evidence that it can be very helpful to people with HIV infection and related health problems. Hydrogen peroxide in bath water is often recommended as an adjunct to other therapies.

Another safe way to enjoy a hydrogen peroxide bath is to spray the body with 3 percent solution of hydrogen peroxide (either diluted from food-grade hydrogen peroxide or the common drugstore variety). Place the hydrogen peroxide in a small spray bottle and apply on the entire body after a shower. The peroxide can then be massaged lightly into the skin. Avoid contact with eyes. The primary disadvantage of this method may affect men with abundant body hair: It will likely turn your hair reddish blond. Those who utilize this method claim that the spray offers the same benefits of a hydrogen peroxide bath; some have reported that it clears up skin blemishes very effectively.

Injection in Joints and Soft-Tissue Trigger Points

Dr. Farr developed and reported the use of 0.03 percent hydrogen peroxide injected into joints and soft tissues. He found that the swelling and inflammation of rheumatoid arthritis and other types of inflammatory arthritis responded quickly to intra-articular injections of hydrogen peroxide. He also found that it was especially effective when injected into osteoarthritic joints such as fingers and knees. Trigger points in muscles and tendons are rapidly relieved with the same type of injection. Some physicians have reported good results in reconstruction of joint surfaces and spaces using hydrogen peroxide injections.[25]

Free Radicals and Hydrogen Peroxide

In chapter 1, the issue of free radicals and oxidation was discussed. Hydrogen peroxide is an activated oxygen species that can break down to liberate free radicals and may sometimes act as a free radical itself. However, it is more often an "intermediate" for the formation of other free radicals like hydroxyl. While hydroxyl is essential for fighting off disease, excessive amounts in the body have been linked to genetic mutations and the destruction of cell membranes. Many physicians believe that hydrogen peroxide is harmful for use in medical therapy because it can lead to the uncontrolled production of free radicals like hydroxyl in the body. However, a closer look at recent findings in the field of free-radical production is needed before reaching such a conclusion.

Dr. Farr found that hydrogen peroxide leads to the formation of hydroxyl radicals only under special circumstances, primarily when ferrous oxide is present. That is why physicians suggest that iron supplements not be taken when hydrogen peroxide is given intravenously or orally and that tap water containing iron not be used to take hydrogen peroxide orally.

When ferrous oxide is not present—which is true most of the time—Dr. Farr has found that hydrogen peroxide is normally converted to oxygen by the enzyme catalase, which renders the hydrogen peroxide beneficial to the body.

The action of catalase on hydrogen peroxide is to add an electron in the presence of hydrogen to pure water and diatomic oxygen. The oxygen is again reduced to superoxide and then to hydrogen peroxide and around the reaction continues. . . . One molecule of catalase can convert millions of molecules of hydrogen peroxide into oxygen and water within seconds and is the body's first line of defense against hydroxyl radical formation.[26]

When taken into the body in small amounts, hydrogen peroxide oxidizes sick, weak, and devitalized cells, while making healthy cells (such as T-cells) stronger and more resistant to oxidation. It also permits the formation of new, healthy cells that are better able to resist disease. This process is essential for healing.

In a later chapter, we discuss the importance of antioxidants (which can easily be found in many popular vegetables and fruits and nutritional supplements) as important adjuncts to bio-oxidative therapy, because they help to keep the body's production of free radicals in check.

As with ozone, there is a wealth of documented evidence that attests to the value of hydrogen peroxide in medical therapy. In part II we explore the latest laboratory and clinical findings that evaluate the use of bio-oxidative therapies to treat many of our most serious health problems.

PART II

BIO-OXIDATIVE THERAPIES IN MEDICINE

Although some of the studies presented in this section are the result of double-blind research (in which neither the patient nor the investigator knows what treatment the patient is receiving), most are of objective and subjective clinical findings based on empirical knowledge or practical experience.

Double-blind trials have become the "gold standard" of scientific research, especially in the United States. The main advantage of this type of research is that complete objectivity is achieved and measurable results are easier to obtain and evaluate. It also prevents the physician from giving any preferential treatment to the patient.

The primary drawback to double-blind studies is that people in need of a valuable treatment may not receive it. In some cases, patients are not permitted to take any other medications (some of which may be life saving) during the trials because the findings of the study might be compromised.

Most German physicians who have done research with medical ozone therapy believe that double-blind studies are immoral. They maintain that ozone is not an experimental drug; it has been used since the First World War and has been proved on millions of patients to be safe and effective. They believe that to deny sick patients a treatment that is likely to relieve their suffering or save their lives is a violation of the Hippocratic oath and an affront to the people who go to them for care. Dr. Joaquim Varro, a physician from Düsseldorf who has worked primarily with cancer patients, shared his views on double-blind studies at the 1983 World Ozone Conference in Washington, D.C.:

> For ethical reasons, and as a practicing physician facing the threat of life in advanced cases, I cannot do a so-called random study or double-blind study. I leave that to science and research with responsibility for such methods. Largely, I adhere to research findings and clinical experiences, and I try to adapt these so that they can be practically applied in my range of activities. As a result, I am able to constructively bring my empirical long-term observations into the medical discussion.[1]

Another problem with double-blind studies is that while they may be a good idea in theory, they do not always work in actual practice. Participants in double-blind trials are known to cheat, especially when their lives are on the line. Several such cases were reported by Paul A. Sergios in *One Boy at War: My Life in the AIDS Underground*. In one instance, he spoke of a double-blind trial for a promising AIDS drug; some participants received an inert sugar pill while others were given the experimental drug. He wrote:

> Numerous patients who were admitted to the trial between February and April 1986 opened their capsules to taste the contents. If the powder tasted bitter, they continued the treatment. If it tasted sweet, they threw the bottle away and rushed to catch a plane to try their luck at getting an actual drug at another site.[2]

Sergios also wrote of his own experience as a participant in another trial for a promising AIDS drug in which he shared half of his pills with another participant to increase their chances of survival in the event that one of them was receiving the experimental medication. When first offered the option of sharing the pills, he said that he felt it was immoral because it could disrupt the trial. His friend replied:

> Immoral? . . . What about their twisted morality in giving half of us a sugar pill for a year or two in order to see how fast we go to our deaths while others get a drug that could potentially save their lives? Not only that—this study prohibits us from taking certain drugs to prevent opportunistic infections. The odds are stacked against *us*.[3]

An unlikely mainstream criticism of double-blind studies was reported on the front page of the September 18, 1997, edition of *The New*

York Times. The article highlighted objection by United States Government scientists and others over National Institutes of Health and Centers for Disease Control and Prevention sponsorship of overseas AIDS studies. In these studies half of 11,211 pregnant women in seven third-world countries were given minimal doses of AZT to determine its ability to prevent HIV infection, while the other half are given dummy pills. It is believed that as a result of this study, more than 1000 infants will contract HIV. The article quotes Dr. Peter Lurie of Public Citizen, an advocacy group, as saying, "We have turned our backs on these mothers and their babies," and cited the Government's own scientists as questioning whether these double-blind studies are ethical.[4]

The decision to use double-blind or random studies involves a number of difficult moral issues that will likely be debated among scientists, physicians, and their patients for years to come. One of my primary goals in this book is to present the evidence, whether it be preliminary, empirical, or the result of double-blind studies. After they see the evidence, it is the task of the readers to either come to their own conclusions or do additional research on their own.

4

CARDIOVASCULAR DISEASES

Physicians have utilized bio-oxidative therapies to treat heart disease and related circulatory problems for over thirty years. Ozone therapy (administered as autohemotherapy, intramuscular injection, intra-arterial injection, or rectal insufflation) and hydrogen peroxide therapy (primarily in the form of intravenous or intra-arterial injection) have been used to treat heart attack, stroke, high blood pressure, cardiac insufficiency, high cholesterol, angina, atherosclerosis, and a wide variety of other problems relating to poor circulation.

In Cuba, ozone therapy has become a routine treatment for patients suffering from angina and heart attacks. During my visit there in January 1994, I met the eighty-year-old mother of Dr. Manuel Gómez, the co-founder of the Department of Ozone. Three years before, Doña Matilde had such severe angina that she could barely get from one room to the other without pain and shortness of breath. After much resistance (she is a very stubborn woman), her son finally persuaded her to undergo three weeks of daily major autohemotherapy, during which the angina completely disappeared. Although Doña Matilde hasn't changed her lifestyle one bit ("I don't like taking long walks."), she has tremendous energy, and her angina symptoms have never returned.

Bio-oxidative therapies work by enhancing blood circulation, which leads to an improvement in the supply of oxygen to tissues. At the same time, hydrogen peroxide and ozone can reactivate the capacity of cells that had previously been deficient to metabolize oxygen more effectively.

In Cuba today, emergency rooms at many major hospitals have an ozone generator to treat victims of heart attack and stroke. In February 1996, Reuters wire service reported that former Nicaraguan president Daniel Ortega Saavedra, the Sandinista leader, who was treated for a heart condition the previous year in Cuba, returned to Havana for a medical check-up. According to the dispatch, the Cuban news agency Prensa Latina said Ortega was receiving a treatment called ozone therapy to purify the blood. It seems that Ortega, a friend of President Fidel Castro, had received ozone therapy for several months beginning in November 1994 after suffering a "silent" heart attack about three months previously.[1]

Ozone and hydrogen peroxide alter the structure of blood and the way it flows through the veins and arteries. The "pile of coins" erythrocyte (mature red blood cell or corpuscle) formation, which is typical of arterial occlusion disease, is reversed through changes in the electrical charge of the erythrocytic membrane. At the same time, the flexibility and elasticity of the erythrocytes are increased, improving the blood's ability to flow through the blood vessels.[2] This increases the supply of life-giving oxygen to the heart and other vital body tissues.

Some of the most important early research in this field was carried out at the New England Medical Center Hospital in Boston. Investigators found that small amounts of hydrogen peroxide alter the way that blood platelets aggregate or come together. Platelets play an important role in the coagulation of blood and the formation of blood clots. In an article published in the journal *Blood,* R. T. Canoso and colleagues concluded: "The generation of peroxide at a site of thrombus [blood clot] formation may alter the development of the thrombus. This alteration could occur via the changes in either aggregation or disaggregation of platelets. . . . "[3]

Other studies at the Upstate Medical Center in Syracuse, New York, and the University of Massachusetts Medical School in Worcester, Massachusetts, later confirmed the role of hydrogen peroxide as a modulator of platelet reactions.[4]

There is also evidence that hydrogen peroxide oxidizes fatty substances like the plaque that adheres to arterial walls. In an article appearing in *Townsend Letter for Doctors,* Dr. Farr writes:

> The oxidative benefit may include the oxidation of lipid material in the vessel wall. The benefit of oxygen saturation of tissue fluid from the oxygen produced by H_2O_2 may be of secondary importance. Cholesterol

and triglycerides become elevated after the intra-arterial injection of H_2O_2. Repeated intra-arterial infusion has been found to remove atheromatous [fatty] plaques and increase elasticity of the blood vessel wall.[5]

In her article "The Biochemical Processes Underlying Ozone Therapy," Renate Viebahn, M.D., addressed the efficacy of medical ozone in improving blood circulation in technical terms:

The so-called circulatory enhancing effects of ozone, as expressed in the form of its being administered intravascularly and intramuscularly, are the result of a direct influence exerted on the oxygen metabolism by the ozone/oxygen mixture applied:

(a) The formation of peroxides from non-saturated fatty acids, and an influence on the rheological properties of the blood,

(b) Activation of the cellular enzymal protection system against peroxides, oxygen and ozone.

(c) Activation of the erythrocytic metabolism and an increase of 2,3-DPG, and

(d) As a fourth factor, a direct influence of the ozone on the redox function of the mitochondrial respiratory chain is considered: this can be demonstrated, for example, by a significant reduction in NADH [an enzyme].

As a total effect, the above properties of ozone bring about a reactivation of the disturbed oxygen metabolism: this is expressed by an increase in the arterial partial oxygen pressure and an enlargement of the arterio-venous PO_2 difference, as well as by an increase in deoxygenating substances producing a greater supply of oxygen to the tissues or by improving the actual processing of oxygen by the system.[6]

We mentioned earlier that bio-oxidative therapies also can activate important enzymes (such as glutathione peroxidase, catalase, and superoxide dismutase) that are involved in free-radical scavenging. An excess of free radicals can contribute to heart disease and other circulatory disturbances.

As we will see in this chapter, the clinical evidence regarding the effectiveness of bio-oxidative therapies in treating different forms of heart disease is well established. Given the fact that heart disease and related circulatory problems are the primary cause of death and disability among adults in this country, it is time to explore the role that bio-oxidative therapies can play in the prevention and treatment of heart disease and related disorders.

Atherosclerosis

Involving the Coronary and Cerebral Vessels

Russian scientists at the Medical Institute in Nizhni Novgorod treated thirty-nine patients suffering from severe atherosclerosis. All patients exhibited symptoms of angina, nine had suffered heart attacks, one had undergone a bypass operation, and two had suffered strokes. Nearly two-thirds of the subjects had cerebral blood supply insufficiency (deficient supply of blood to the brain), and one-quarter had a condition called discirculatory encephalopathy, causing impaired circulation in the brain.

Over twenty days of treatment, ozonated sodium chloride was given intravenously five times a day. By the end of the study, angina attacks decreased from an average of 6.1 to 2.5 per day. Doses of nitroglycerine were reduced. Tolerance to physical load increased in 82.1 percent of the patients. Of those suffering from repolarization impairments (defined by *Taber's Cyclopedic Medical Dictionary* as "reestablishment of a polarized state in a muscle or nerve fiber following contraction or conduction of a nerve impulse"), 51.1 percent recovered completely. In addition, within the group, cholesterol levels dropped 48 percent and triglyceride levels fell 53 percent.

These favorable results led the researchers to conclude that ozone therapy should be considered an effective method for treatment of atherosclerosis in the medical clinic.[7]

An important study on the effects of ozone on blood in heart attack patients was undertaken by scientists at the Ozone Research Center in Cuba. They noted that patients who suffer from heart attack (cardiac infarction) show a decrease in glutathione peroxidase and superoxide dismutase activities, which are beginners in the scavenger processes of lipid peroxide and superoxide radicals, respectively. The goal of the study was to investigate the effects of endovenous ozone therapy (i.e., major autohemotherapy) on serum lipid pattern and on antioxidant defense system, such as the glutathione redox in the blood of twenty-two male patients from forty-six to seventy-six years of age who had suffered a heart attack between three months and one year before the study. The patients were given autohemo-therapy once per weekday over a period of three weeks for a total of fifteen treatments.

At the end of the course of treatment, researchers observed a statistically significant decrease in plasma total cholesterol and low-density lipoprotein ("bad" cholesterol). In addition, biologically significant increases on erythrocyte glutathione peroxidase and glucose 6-phosphate dehydrogenase activities were found. There was no change in plasma lipid peroxidation level. The researchers concluded that "endovenous ozone therapy in patients with myocardial infarction has a beneficial effect on blood lipid metabolism, provoking the activation of antioxidant protection system."[8]

Involving the Extremities

In the early 1990s, researchers at the Department of Gerontology, Geriatry and Metabolic Diseases at the Second University of Naples in Italy compared the effectiveness of hyperbaric oxygen and oxygen–ozone therapy in treating patients suffering from peripheral occlusive arterial disease (POAD). In this study, researchers investigated the influence of these treatments on medical parameters that play an important role in the origin and the clinical course of arteriosclerosis. Two groups of fifteen patients suffering from POAD were assigned at random either to a cycle of hyperbaric oxygen therapy or oxygen– ozone therapy. Blood was tested to evaluate blood viscosity, erythrocyte filterability, hematocrit value, fibrinogen concentration, and thrombin time, which are all used to determine the nature and extent of the disease. The researchers found that the oxygen–ozone therapy brought about a significant increase of erythrocyte filterability and a significant decrease of blood viscosity, showing that they help relieve symptoms of POAD. In contrast, hyperbaric oxygen therapy did not produce any significant change in the blood. The researchers concluded, "The increase of lipid perioxidation, proved by raised malonyldialdehyde plasma levels, seems a likely mechanism involved in the hemorrheologic effects of O_2-O_3 therapy."[9]

A major study on the effects of medical ozone on patients suffering from symptoms of atherosclerosis in the extremities was undertaken by the Viennese surgeon Ottokar Rokitansky at a large Vienna hospital. During the early 1980s, he evaluated 232 patients whose symptoms fit the last three of four categories of the disease as classified by the French heart specialist G. Fontaine:

Stage I: rapid tiring, exhaustion, sensation of coldness
Stage II: latent pain(s), intermittent lameness or limping
Stage III: pains when lying down at night or at rest
Stage IV: gangrene

In the third and fourth stages, amputation of fingers, toes, or limbs is often necessary.

The participants in the study were divided into two groups of roughly similar ages and symptoms: In Group 1, an oxygen–ozone mixture was added to the patients' blood by intra-arterial injection. In addition, ozone gas was applied within a plastic bag that surrounded the affected limb (as described in chapter 2). Group 2 consisted of a control group of 140 who received traditional vasodilation therapy—medication designed to open up blood vessels.

Dr. Rokitansky reported marked clinical improvement in up to 80 percent of the patients suffering from Stage II of the disease who received ozone therapy, as compared to 44 percent of the patients receiving traditional therapy. At-rest pains disappeared for 70 percent of the people in Stage III who received ozone, as compared to 39 percent of the control group. The Stage IV patients, who were all hospitalized, had a 50 percent cure rate of the ulcers and soft-tissue gangrene, which reduced their time in the hospital; by contrast, similar results were achieved by only 28.6 percent of the controls. The rate of upper thigh amputations declined from 15 percent to 10 percent for the Stage III patients and from 50 percent to 27 percent for patients with gangrene (Stage IV) who received ozone (table 4.1).[10]

In 1988, a study was done at the National Institute of Angiology and Vascular Surgery in Havana on sixty patients suffering from severe atherosclerosis. Primary symptoms included blocked blood circulation to their extremities, primarily the feet. The patients were divided into two groups so that the age range and symptoms were similar. Half received ten daily sessions of either autohemotherapy with oxygen and ozone or intra-arterial injections of oxygen and ozone. The control group was given traditional medical treatment.

By the end of the ten days, 73.4 percent of the fifteen patients with less severe atherosclerosis treated with ozone exhibited marked improvement,

Table 4.1. Therapy Cases Compared

Stage	Number of Subjects		Marked Improvement %		Some Improvement %		Deterioration or no improvement %	
	1	2	1	2	1	2	1	2
II	105	73	80.0	43.8	11.4	19.2	8.5	37.0
III	72	46	70.8	39.1	19.4	17.4	9.7	43.5
IV	55	21	50.9	28.6	21.8	19.0	27.3	54.0

Source: Ottokar Rokitansky, "The Clinical Effects and Biochemistry of Ozone Therapy in Peripheral Arterial Coronary Disturbances," Medical Applications of Ozone, edited by Julius LaRaus (Norwalk, Conn.: The International Ozone Association, Pan American Committee, 1983), 53.

while the condition of 20 percent deteriorated. In contrast, 40 percent of the control group of fifteen improved, while 53 percent got worse. The fifteen patients who suffered from more serious symptoms (which included severe pain, gangrene, and ischemic ulcers) who were treated with ozone showed good results. Sixty percent experienced clinical improvement, while only 26 percent of the control group of fifteen improved. Six patients (40 percent) receiving ozone got worse as compared to eleven patients (73 percent) in the control group.[11]

In 1989, a study was undertaken in Poland by Dr. J. Sroczynski and colleagues at the Katedry i Kliniki Chorob Wewnetrznych i Zawodowych SI. AM, a research hospital specializing in internal and occupational diseases. Ozone was administered intra-arterially to fifty subjects suffering from arteriosclerotic ischemia of the lower extremities and forty-one subjects with diabetes mellitus. Serum lipid concentrations were examined before and after the course of treatment. Researchers reported that the group with arteriosclerotic ischemia experienced a "significant" decrease in blood cholesterol level. At the same time, the patients suffering from diabetes showed a significant reduction of LDL (or "bad") cholesterol. In both groups total lipid level serum was decreased. According to an abstract of this article poorly translated into English, the researchers concluded that "ozone therapy set back the arteriosclerosis progress, normalized some parameters of lipid metabolism and improved

HDL to LDL cholesterol fractions relationship."[12]

Two other Polish studies carried out in the early 1990s revealed the positive effects of ozone therapy on circulatory problems of the lower limbs. In the first study, investigators at the Katedry i Zakladu Biofizyki Sl. examined fifty-three patients with occlusive arteriosclerosis of the lower limbs. Blood and plasma viscosity, total lipids, triglycerides, total cholesterol, free fatty acids, fibrinogen, lipid-gram, and hematocrit levels were determined both prior to and after a course of ozone therapy. At the same time, intermittent claudication distance was measured, which evaluated lameness or difficulty in walking. The results were very positive: After ozone therapy, all patients showed a significant prolongation of the distance walked painlessly. In addition, there was a marked reduction in blood and plasma viscosity as well as the decrease in total cholesterol after therapy with ozone.[13]

The second study, which was coordinated by Dr. Sroczynski as a follow-up to his earlier research, was undertaken at the Katedry i Kliniki Chorob Wennetrznych i Zawodoych, another medical school clinic. In this study, doctors investigated the value of intra-arterial ozone injections in the treatment of atherosclerotic ischemia. Ten injections of ozone and oxygen were administered into the femoral arteries of fifty patients suffering from atherosclerotic ischemia of the lower extremities over a period of several weeks. The same treatment was given to forty-nine diabetic patients suffering from similar symptoms. All patients were assessed clinically with standard medical tests, including the "ankle–arm index" and measurement of intermittent claudication distance prior to and after the treatment. The results showed a significant improvement in both groups as measured by an increase in the ankle–arm index, as well as a twofold prolongation of the intermittent claudication distance. The researchers concluded that treating atherosclerotic ischemia of the lower extremities with ozone is both "valuable and safe."[14]

Researchers at the Ozone Therapy Center in Nizhni Novgorod, Russia, also studied the effect of ozone therapy on atherosclerotic vessel disorders of the lower extremities and announced their findings at the Twelfth World Congress of the International Ozone Association in 1995. Working in cooperation with the Nizhegorodski Regional Hospital of War Veterans, 132 war invalids, sixty-two to eighty-four years of age, suffering from III–IV grade peripheral circulation disorders of the lower extremities were observed.

Although all had been receiving traditional medical care over the years, none of the patients was able to walk for a distance of more than 150–200 meters. All experienced chronic pain in the calf muscles and had cold lower legs and feet. Eleven war veterans suffered from crus and femur wounds of forty-seven to fifty years standing, while eight patients had been afflicted with frostbite during the Second World War. Thirty-one of the patients had circulation problems accompanied by chronic trophic ulcers.

Different types of ozone therapy were administered to patients who were divided into three groups depending on symptoms. The first group were given eight to ten intravenous injections of ozone-saturated rheopolyglucin solutions (rheamacrodex). The second group received intravenous ozone injections combined with subcutaneous injections of ozone and oxygen. The third group were given a course of three to four autohemotherapy treatments in addition to the therapies above. Patients with trophic ulcers were given external ozonation through the plastic bag method described in chapter 2.

By the end of the courses of treatment virtually all patients exhibited a "significant improvement in their well-being" with warming of the extremities and complete relief of muscle cramps. There was also an average ten- to fifteenfold increase in walking distance. The trophic ulcers all shrank from 2 to 4 cm^2 daily during and after treatment, eliminating the need for surgery. The researchers concluded that ozone therapy (especially the combination of the three types of ozone therapies) was "highly effective" in the treatment of peripheral circulatory disorders of the lower extremities, especially in people advanced in age.[15]

A Cuban study involved seventy-two elderly nondiabetic patients with obliterant atherosclerosis, compounded by intermittent claudication, or severe pain in the calf muscles while walking. The patients were randomly divided into four groups. Three of the groups were treated with ozone: one group with major autohemotherapy, another via intramuscular injection, and the last with rectal insufflation. Members of the fourth group of patients (the control group) were given conventional medical treatment. Members of the first three groups who were treated with ozone showed little difference among them; however, the three groups showed considerable improvement when compared to members of the control group. The claudication distance in the treadmill increased to 2.5 km/hr. Ankle–arm pressure rates showed a significant difference as well, which corresponds to the Polish findings mentioned earlier. Patients reported that of all methods of ozone application, rectal insufflation was the least uncomfortable.[16]

Heart Defects (with Infectious Endocarditis)

An unusual study was carried out at the Interregional Cardiosurgical Center at Nizhni Novgorod in Russia on patients undergoing heart surgery whose cases were complicated by endocarditis, an inflammation of the membrane lining the heart. When endocarditis was present, over one-quarter of the heart patients typically died during or after surgery.

During the operations undertaken as part of the study, the patients' hearts were bathed in ozonated cardioplegic solutions, which are designed to stop the heart. These solutions were infused with ozone before application. A heart–lung machine circulated the blood (to which a mixture of oxygen and ozone was added) during the operation.

The results showed that the death rate from complications of infectious endocarditis fell from an average of 26.6 percent to only 4.2 percent.[17]

Hypercholesteremia (Excessive Cholesterol)

Some of the most important research in the field of bio-oxidative therapies, particularly in the areas of heart disease and cancer, took place at Baylor University Medical Center in Dallas in the early 1960s. In one study, Dr. J. W. Finney and his colleagues studied the ability of hydrogen peroxide to remove cholesterol and other fats from the arteries. They based this early research on postmortem studies of the arteries of cancer patients who had received intra-arterial hydrogen peroxide (as an adjunct to irradiation therapy) for a period of four to sixteen weeks in the late stages of their disease. The blood vessels of a similar group of cancer patients who did not receive hydrogen peroxide were studied for comparison.

When the blood vessel samples were analyzed, it was found that the patients receiving hydrogen peroxide had an approximately 50 percent reduction in total lipids (fats) in the area that had been infused with hydrogen peroxide.[18]

A study at the Medical and Surgical Research Center in Havana a quarter century later (see p. 68) involved twenty-two men between the ages of forty-six and seventy-two who had had heart attacks. All patients had elevated levels of total cholesterol as well as low-density lipoproteins, the most dangerous form of cholesterol. The only treatment given during the study consisted of fifteen sessions of autohemotherapy with ozone.

After five treatments, cholesterol levels had fallen an average of 5.5 percent, and by the end of the treatment period of fifteen sessions, the levels of cholesterol in the blood had fallen by an average of 9.7 percent. Levels of low-density lipoproteins had decreased 15.4 percent after five sessions of autohemotherapy and 19.8 percent by the fifteenth session.

The researchers concluded, "Endovenous ozone therapy has beneficial effects on [the] lipid pattern of patients that have suffered myocardial infarction [heart attack]; and accompanied by an effective stimulation of [the] antioxidant enzyme system."[19]

Hypoxia

Another of the Baylor studies found that hydrogen peroxide can provide oxygen for the anoxic or ischemic heart, as well as help normalize cardiac arrhythmias and reverse cardiac arrest. Dr. Harold C. Urschel Jr., who was involved in much of the Baylor research, expounded on these findings in the journal *Diseases of the Chest:*

> Hydrogen peroxide releases dissolved oxygen equivalent to that found in solutions under oxygen at 3–8 atmosphere pressure [i.e., hyperbaric oxygen]. H_2O_2 administration does not require lung transport. It can be given continuously over long periods of time, it can be administered by a single physician without expensive equipment and large teams, and it avoids compression–decompression hazards, as well as central nervous system and pulmonary toxicity.[20]

Additional research at Baylor University focused on the ability of hydrogen peroxide to protect the heart during ischemic episodes of heart attacks. Using pigs as subjects, Dr. Finney and his colleagues found that diluted solutions of hydrogen peroxide were able to keep the heart functioning in spite of an ischemic episode. By adding dimethyl sulfate (DMSO) to the hydrogen peroxide mixture, the scientists discovered that the new mixture "will afford more protection [to the heart] than either reagent alone."[21] It is interesting to note that the Baylor studies, which were supported at first by a large pharmaceutical company, have experienced little or no clinical follow-up.

Similar results have been achieved with ozone. Dr. S. P. Peretyagin of the Medical Institute in Nizhni Novgorod performed a clinical study of how ozone can increase the flow of oxygen through the blood vessels.[22] This increased delivery of oxygen to the heart and brain is why in many of the larger Cuban hospitals, ozone therapy is routinely used in emergency rooms and intensive care units for patients who come to the hospital suffering from heart attacks or strokes. The ozone provides the heart and brain with the vital oxygen they need by enabling the blood to flow more freely through the circulatory system.

Ischemic Heart Disease

As in the United States and Canada, ischemic heart disease is a leading health problem in Russia. Primary symptoms of ischemic heart disease (IHD) are stable and unstable angina pectoris, involving pain and pressure around the heart due to insufficient blood to the heart. An attack may last from several seconds to several minutes.

A group of physicians from the regional Diagnostic Center in Nizhni Novgorod studied the efficiency of ozone therapy in patients suffering from IHD. A group of eighty-five adults were chosen for the study: Eighty had symptoms of stable II–III stenocardia, which is a type of angina pectoris. The other five had progressive angina pectoris. Oxygen and ozone was administered intravenously in a saline solution and as rectal insufflations over a three- to four-week period. Patients were carefully monitored through observation of angina attacks and nitroglycerine use, tolerance to physical exercise, electrocardiogram readings, and echocardioscopy.

After the course of treatment, researchers found that chest pains were completely controlled in forty-six of the eighty patients (58 percent) with stable stenocardia, while thirty others (37.5 percent) reported fewer attacks of pain. Four patients showed no improvement. All of the patients suffering from progressive angina showed marked improvement, with a significant reduction of coronary insufficiency symptoms.[23]

Ischemic Cerebrovascular Disease

Ischemic cerebrovascular disease involves a blocking of the blood supply to the brain, often incapacitating patients both mentally and physically. This disease is a leading cause of death among the elderly in many of the industrialized nations of the world.

A Cuban study regarding the ability of ozone to improve the health status of older adults suffering from ischemic cerebrovascular disease was carried out at the Geriatric Complex of the Salvador Allende Hospital in Havana. A group of 120 was chosen for the study.

Extensive physical, neurological (including CT scan and EEGs), multidimensional psychological, and psychomotor tests were given before and after treatment. Special attention was devoted to the patients' mental condition, ability to participate in daily activities, ability to administer their own medications, and social interaction with friends and family. Patients were then classified into three standardized groups according to their symptoms: Forty-eight (40 percent) were in an "acute" phase of the disease; forty-two (35 percent) were in an "ancient" phase; and thirty (25 percent) were classified as being in the "chronic" phase of the disease. Treatment consisted of fifteen sessions of ozone therapy given through rectal insufflation over a period of three weeks.

The results were impressive. The mental condition of all acute-phase patients improved by the end of therapy, along with 91 percent of those in the ancient phase and 67 percent in the chronic phase. By the same token, the physical condition of all acute-phase patients improved, while improvement took place in 67 percent of those in the ancient phase and 47 percent of those in the chronic phase of the disease. Post-therapy tests revealed that the subject's ability to participate in daily life situations improved in all of the acute-phase patients, 95 percent of those in the ancient phase, and 80 percent of those in the chronic phase.

The researchers concluded:

1. Ozone therapy, in the way and doses applied, produced significant improvement in the group of patients with cerebrovascular disease of the ischemic type, being more effective the faster the therapy begins.

2. The initial clinical state improved in 88 percent of the patients treated, obtaining better results in those in the acute phase.

3. In the multidimensional evaluation, all parameters measured improved, especially daily life activities.

4. No adverse reactions were reported during the treatment.[24]

Those results have led the physicians at the Salvador Allende Hospital to use ozone therapy on all patients who enter the facility for the treatment of ischemic cerebrovascular disease.

Stroke

Physicians have found that early intervention of ozone applications can help reduce the severity of symptoms of people who suffer a stroke. This is believed to be partly due to ozone's ability to increase the level of adenosine triphosphate (ATP) to tissues, improve blood circulation, and aid in the release of oxygen to the body's cells. Ozone generators can be found in many hospital emergency rooms in Cuba, where they are used primarily to treat patients suffering from heart attack and stroke.

One of the few clinical studies of stroke patients and ozone therapy was carried out by Gerd Wasser, M.D., of the Wasser Clinic in Germany. He studied forty-five patients who had recently suffered from acute brain stroke. Although patients already received primary treatment at the hospital, none received the full course of traditional medical care.

Three different types of poststroke syndrome were established:

Type 1: All functions (including fine motoric movement) is reestablished. Sensory failures are possible but not obvious at first glance.

Type 2: Patients did not restore fine motoric movement, but were able to regain a basic level of motoric nerve transmission.

Type 3: Patients were confined to bed due to paralysis.

After a course of treatment with ozone therapy, the results were very encouraging. Forty of the forty-five patients moved into Type 1 and five patients were classified in Type 2. None of the patients remained paralyzed, and none of them died. This is far better than the average outcome for stroke patients, which normally includes a 30 percent death rate. Of the survivors, approximately 55 percent remain handicapped and 15 percent need total care for twenty-four hours a day.

In his presentation at the Twelfth Ozone World Congress in Lille,

France, in 1995, Dr. Wasser recommended that ozone therapy be applied as soon as possible after the stroke occurs: "The total dosage should reach 3000 micrograms of O_3. In the following days the same dosage will be given once a day. Edema–related paralysis disappeared in all cases within 10 minutes. Relapses are very rare and can receive the same treatment described above."[25]

Despite the tremendous promise that bio-oxidative therapies offer to patients suffering from heart and circulatory disease, little research is being done in this country to study ozone and hydrogen peroxide. No studies have been sponsored by the American Heart Association, the National Institutes of Health, the Centers for Disease Control and Prevention, or any other major organization in this country to scientifically evaluate bio-oxidative therapies among large groups of people.

By the same token, no studies have evaluated the preventive effects of regular ozone or hydrogen peroxide treatment among people who may be genetically predisposed to heart attack or for individuals who are otherwise at risk for heart disease or stroke.

5

CANCER

Cancer has been treated with hydrogen peroxide and ozone therapy for decades. The rationale behind the use of bio-oxidative therapies to treat cancer is based on three important discoveries.

The first discovery was made by Nobel Prize winner Dr. Otto Warburg, director of the Max Planck Institute for Cell Physiology in Berlin. He confirmed (at a meeting of fellow Nobel laureates by the shores of Lake Constance, Germany, in 1966) that the key precondition for the development of cancer is a lack of oxygen at the cellular level.[1]

The second important factor was addressed by another Nobel Prize winner, Dr. James D. Watson, the codiscoverer of the DNA double helix. He found that "among the most useful carcinogenic agents known at present are several viruses."[2] Thus, the development of cancer was known to have a viral component that was not recognized before.

The third discovery, which was first reported by Dr. Joaquim Varro of Germany, in 1974, revealed a peroxide intolerance in tumor cells, suggesting that ozone and hydrogen peroxide may induce metabolic inhibition in certain types of cancerous growths.[3] This was not confirmed in an English-language publication until 1980, when an article by Dr. Frederick Sweet and his colleagues in the journal *Science* introduced laboratory evidence proving that ozone selectively inhibits the growth of cancer cells.[4]

One of the physicians to offer tentative support for the use of bio-oxidative therapies in treating cancer years ago was Boguslaw Lipinski, M.D., of the Boston Cardiovascular Health Center and the Tufts University School of Medicine:

> Preliminary clinical studies indicate that oxidative therapy might produce desirable results in cancer treatment. . . . Exposure of patients' blood in vitro to ozone and subsequent injection is a medical procedure used for a successful treatment of cancer in one Swiss clinic [the famous Roka Clinic] since 1960. . . . Although these preliminary findings do not constitute proof in themselves, they may certainly encourage clinical researchers and practitioners to try this unorthodox but apparently promising modality.[5]

In the following pages, we examine some of the laboratory and clinical evidence that lends support to the concept that ozone and hydrogen peroxide can assist in the treatment of cancer, either alone or as an adjunct to traditional or alternative cancer therapies.

Hydrogen Peroxide Studies

Early cancer research at the Baylor University Medical Center in Dallas was begun in the early 1960s by Dr. J. W. Finney and his associates. One of the first articles discussing their findings was published in the *Southern Medical Journal* in March 1962 and spoke of the value of hydrogen peroxide as an adjunct to radiation therapy for treating cancer. "The Use of Hydrogen Peroxide as a Source of Oxygen in a Regional Intra-arterial Infusion System" revealed that cancer cells become more sensitive to irradiation in the presence of increased oxygen tension produced by hydrogen peroxide. Phases I and II of the study involved laboratory animals. In Phase III, doses of hydrogen peroxide diluted in water were administered intra-arterially to patients suffering from a variety of carcinomas. The researchers noted increased regional oxygenation, which led them to believe that there is an "increased therapeutic ratio" in malignant tumors receiving radiation when oxygen levels of the affected area are increased with hydrogen peroxide.[6]

A related Baylor University cancer study (this time with large, inoperable abdominal tumors) using intra-arterial hydrogen peroxide and irradiation was undertaken. The researchers wanted to see if hydrogen peroxide could shrink the tumors and make them amenable to surgery. Two of the three patients experienced a shrinkage of their tumors and underwent successful operations to remove them. The third patient experienced no changes after four weeks and was sent home to die. To everyone's surprise, however, he began to improve over the next several months, and the tumor began shrinking considerably. The doctors later removed the shrunken tumor with no complications. In their article in the journal *Cancer*, the researchers concluded:

> The resection of this tumor apparently was made possible by presurgical medium dose irradiation associated with regional oxygenation by the intra-arterial infusion of a solution of hydrogen peroxide into the abdominal aorta. The findings in 2 other patients with intra-abdominal tumors have been summarized in regard to the usefulness of intra-arterial hydrogen peroxide procedures. The findings justify further investigation in these areas.[7]

Another early study concerning the value of hydrogen peroxide as a complementary therapy for cancer was conducted in Japan in 1966 at the Tottori University School of Medicine. Fifteen patients suffering from maxillary cancer (cancer of the nasal cavity and/or jaw) were given intra-arterial infusions of hydrogen peroxide daily for ten days, followed by daily injection of mitomycin C (Mutamycin), an antibiotic showing antitumor activity. A control group of twenty-nine received the anticancer agent alone.

Operations were then done to remove and analyze the tumors. Of the fifteen patients treated with hydrogen peroxide and Mutamycin, eight showed almost a complete disappearance of the tumor, while six experienced a partial reduction. One had little change. The changes involved either an actual shrinking of the tumor or a softening of a hard tumor, described by the researchers (in a way that must be unique to Japanese doctors) as having the texture of tofu, or bean curd. Of the patients who received the anticancer drug alone, six experienced complete disappearance, twenty-one had partial reduction, and two showed no response.

In their summary, the researchers wrote: "Enhancement of the anticancer agent was observed. We have also proven clinically that the method [does not] cause danger in each individual patient."[8]

The antitumor effects of hydrogen peroxide were also studied by Dr. Carl F. Nathan and Dr. Zanvil A. Cohn at Rockefeller University in New York City. In their article, published in the *Journal of Experimental*

Medicine in 1979, they wrote, "Hydrogen peroxide contributes to the lysis [destruction] of tumor cells by macrophages [immune cells that devour pathogens and other intruders] and granulocytes [white blood cells that act as scavengers to combat infection] in vitro." (In a later in vivo experiment, they found that eight milligrams of hydrogen peroxide killed more than 90 percent of P338 lymphoma cells.)[9]

At the same time, their research led them to conclude that hydrogen peroxide could exert a "direct anti-tumor effect in vivo and thereby prolong the survival of the host [the patient]." Like the Japanese, they added that "hydrogen peroxide can synergize in vivo with certain anti-tumor drugs already in use."[10]

The results of a more recent study undertaken at the University of California at Irvine on the ability of hydrogen peroxide to kill cancer cells associated with Hodgkin's disease were published in the June 1989 issue of *Cancer*. Dr. Michael K. Samoszuk and his colleagues from the Department of Pathology took cell suspensions from twenty-three lymph nodes of living patients and subjected them to a low concentration of hydrogen peroxide. They found that a substantial killing of the infected cells took place after only fifteen minutes of incubation. The researchers observed that "peroxidase in Hodgkin's disease sensitizes the tumor cells to killing by low levels of hydrogen peroxide" and concluded:

> The significance of our observation is that it provides a rationale for investigating new therapeutic modalities designed specifically to deliver cytotoxic quantities of hydrogen peroxide to Hodgkin's disease.[11]

Research with Ozone

As in the hydrogen peroxide studies, the first cancer research in the United States concerning ozone therapy involved laboratory animals. One of the first preliminary American studies on the effects of ozone on mammary carcinomas was reported in the early 1980s by Dr. Migdalia Arnan and Lee E. DeVries at the Northern Dutchess Hospital in Rhinebeck, New York. Mice with mammary carcinomas were injected with a mixture of ozone and oxygen, while the mice in the control group were untreated. The tumors died in the mice receiving ozone. However, the dead tumor tissues were not removed, which was believed to present a burden to the tissue macrophages, suppressing the immune system of the ozonated mice. Nevertheless, the group of mice receiving ozone survived thirty to forty-eight days longer than the control group.[12]

Also as with hydrogen peroxide, it is believed that the anticancer effects of medical ozone are connected to its ability to induce the body's release of tumor necrosis factor, which is involved in killing cancerous tumors. In an article published in *Lymphokine and Cytokine Research* in 1991, Drs. Luana Paulesu, Enrico Luzzi, and Velio Bocci of the Department of General Physiology at the University of Siena in Italy discussed their experiments measuring tumor necrosis factor in ozonated blood. They found that most of the tumor necrosis factor was released immediately after ozonation took place. They called their findings "novel and interesting" and thought they could help explain the beneficial clinical effects of autohemotherapy that had been utilized in Europe for decades. The researchers concluded, "This is of obvious importance not only for the treatment of viral diseases but also for immunodepressed and tumor bearing patients."[13]

As mentioned earlier, the first time the possible effectiveness of ozone as a cancer treatment for humans was reported in a major scientific periodical was in the journal *Science* in 1980 by Dr. Frederick Sweet and his associates at the Washington University School of Medicine in St. Louis. Using in vitro studies, they found that the growth of human cancer cells from lung, breast, and uterine tumors was selectively inhibited by ozone given in a dose of 0.3 to 0.8 parts per million over a period of eight days. Exposure to ozone at 0.8 parts per million inhibited cancer cell growth more than 90 percent and controlled cell growth to less than 50 percent. They also noted that there was no growth inhibition of normal cells, which they felt was due to the fact that "cancer cells are less able to compensate for the oxidative burden of ozone than normal cells."[14]

One of the first reports on the successful use of ozone therapy with actual patients was by the German surgeon Joachim Varro at the Sixth World Ozone Conference in 1983. Dr. Varro is considered one of the pioneers in the use of medical ozone to treat cancer, and his work is admired around the world.

Dr. Varro believes that cancer is not the result of an outside infection but has its source in the body itself:

> The malignant tumor is not an exogenous foreign body like a virus or bacteria, but rather a substance of the body proper, consisting of organic cells and behaving autonomously as a foreign body only because of

misinformation in its growth impulses. It has removed itself from the orderly principles of the organism as a whole. Thus, the tumor is not actually the cause of metabolic chaos but should be seen as the end product of a misguided prior pathophysiological development.[15]

In his article, Dr. Varro did not provide statistical data. Since many of his patients came to his office as a last resort, many of them had undergone surgery, chemotherapy, and radiation. For those reasons, he believed that statistical evaluation would be difficult to document. However, among his patients, he noted that ozone therapy had a marked effect. Patients experienced increased appetite, greater strength, higher rates of physical activity, and a reduction in pain. He offered his clinical evaluation of the patients who had undergone ozone–oxygen therapy:

1. Side effects and after effects of surgery and radiation can frequently be diminished and even completely eliminated; the same applies to cytostatic consequences of chemotherapy [which prevents the growth and proliferation of cells].

2. The patients are free of metastasis and tumor relapses for remarkably long periods of time.

3. The survival time could be prolonged, far exceeding the usual dubious prognoses, even in cases of inoperability, radiation resistance, or chemotherapy non-tolerance, and with improved quality of life.

4. Most patients who had undergone the combination therapy *shortly* after surgery and radiation could return full time to their occupations.[16]

Current Therapies

At the Hospital Santa Monica in Mexico, founded by Kurt W. Donsbach and believed to be the largest hospital providing holistic health care in the world, intravenous hydrogen peroxide is used extensively to treat cancer. Thousands of patients have come to the hospital as a last resort when traditional medical therapy failed them, and many have experienced complete recovery. In his book *Wholistic Cancer Therapy* Dr. Donsbach has the following to say about the therapeutic use of food-grade hydrogen peroxide:

1. Cancer cells are less virulent and may even be destroyed by the presence of a high oxygen environment.

2. Hydrogen peroxide given by transfusion and orally has the ability to increase the oxygen content of the blood stream which will increase the oxygen environment of the cancer cell.

3. Clinical evidence has overwhelmingly convinced me that the use of hydrogen peroxide is a valuable adjunct in the treatment of cancer.[17]

In addition to hydrogen peroxide, Dr. Donsbach utilizes vitamin therapy, mineral therapy, hyperthermia, and other natural modalities during the patient's course of treatment. When administering daily doses of intravenous hydrogen peroxide, he includes dimethyl sulfoxide, a solvent used by physicians primarily to facilitate absorption of medicines through the skin. Dr. Donsbach found that DMSO helps mitigate the irritation that some patients experience with hydrogen peroxide. In addition, he believes DMSO to be a cancer treatment in its own right and also credits it with being able to retard the growth of bacteria, viruses, and fungi and reduce inflammation and swelling. He gives daily infusions of hydrogen peroxide and DMSO to all patients throughout their courses of treatment at the hospital.

Dr. Donsbach and his associates also use medical ozone at the Hospital Santa Monica, although to a lesser extent than hydrogen peroxide. In his book *Oxygen–Peroxide–Ozone*, he wrote:

Recent advances in ozone manufacture and technology have created a great interest on my part in using humidified ozone by rectal insufflation. The methodology allows repeated treatment during the day without invasive procedures such as required to give an intravenous infusion. The rectal tip is introduced and a thirty-second burst of humidified ozone is injected into the rectum, yielding about one-half liter. It is very painless and the reports I have seen indicate a higher concentration of oxygen can be achieved in the bloodstream by this method than injecting the ozone directly into the bloodstream. Our patients love it because there is almost always a feeling of well-being immediately after the treatment. We use this up to three times per day in critical patients. This treatment method is unique in that it avoids the intestinal cramps that injecting dry ozone into the rectum causes.[18]

I asked Dr. Donsbach for statistics regarding the number of people cured of cancer at Hospital Santa Monica. He replied that statistics are an illusive factor but added:

Approximately 70 percent of our patients are alive three years after their first visit to our facility. Some are cured, some are in remission and some are slowly dying. However, very few of these patients had more than months to live according to their doctors when they arrived. But what kind of statistics are these? We see a significant percentage of our patients become totally and completely cured as documented by medical diagnostic standards.[19]

Dr. Horst Kief has been using autohomologous immunotherapy (AHIT) extensively to treat a variety of cancers. During my visit to his clinic in December 1993, I observed a woman receiving treatment for breast cancer, which had recurred after traditional medical treatment. Through the use of oral AHIT and AHIT injections applied around the infected part of the breast, the patient experienced a rapid remission. Jon Greenberg, M.D., a former associate of Dr. Kief, reported that the long-term remission rate for cancer patients receiving AHIT at the Kief Clinic is 60 percent, with another 20 percent of patients experiencing improvement.[20]

In 1988, Dr. Kief studied thirty-one patients suffering from a variety of malignancies, including carcinomas, lymphomas, a sarcoma, and a kidney tumor. Most had received chemotherapy and radiation, without long-term success. AHIT was given daily over a four-month period.

The results showed that after four weeks of AHIT, levels of gamma interferon increased by 700 to 900 percent. Gamma interferon is a protein found when cells are exposed to viruses; noninfected cells exposed to interferon are protected against viral infection. Overall, Kief observed dramatic subjective improvement in patients, including a decrease of pain in 70 percent and increases in vitality in 90 percent of the patients using AHIT.[21]

During my interview with Dr. Kief, one of the participants in that study, a sixty-two-year-old man, happened by the clinic for a routine examination. In 1988 he was diagnosed with immunocytoma Stage IVb, a particularly lethal cancer that involves the lymph nodes. The oncologists who treated him held out no hope for his recovery. After eleven months of AHIT, the patient experienced a complete remission, which continued when I met him four years later.[22]

Ongoing research points to the suitability of medical ozone and hydrogen peroxide for cancer treatment. An article published in the British magazine *New Scientist* discussed findings presented at an April 1994 meeting of the American Association of Cancer Researchers in San Francisco that oxygen can be an important part of tumor treatment. It appears that tumors have regions that are starved of oxygen, which results when blood vessels grow haphazardly inside a developing cancer. The article reported that Dr. Beverly Teicher of the prestigious Dana-Farber Cancer Institute in Boston told the meeting that this lack of oxygen was hampering treatment by protecting the tumor against conventional therapies such as radiation and chemotherapy. By increasing the oxygen levels in the tumor, conventional therapy can be more successful. Although the methods highlighted in the meetings included a synthetic blood substitute, ozone and hydrogen peroxide have similar applications.

The article added that clinical trials on patients with superficial tumors, such as melanomas, are promising and mentioned that other cancer therapies have been designed to exploit the hypoxia at Stanford University, using anticancer drugs designed to work in almost anaerobic conditions. These findings appear to confirm both Dr. Warburg's conclusions and the early Baylor University studies that link cancerous tumors to low oxygen levels and the ability of bio-oxidative therapies to destroy tumors by increasing oxygen tension in malignant cells.[23]

It is hoped that more clinical studies can be made with cancer patients treated by ozone and hydrogen peroxide, but that will probably not happen. Given the life-threatening nature of cancer, few people will agree to undergo a double-blind study in which they may have to discontinue another therapy that may be keeping them alive. In addition, the value of bio-oxidative therapies is rarely witnessed in patients who have never received other cancer treatments, since most patients seek out therapy with ozone or hydrogen peroxide after chemotherapy, radiation, and surgery have failed them.

Despite those considerations, there is growing clinical and laboratory evidence that these therapies are of value. Tens of thousands of European patients are becoming cancer free thanks to ozone therapy, while hundreds of Americans are beginning to understand the value of hydrogen peroxide and ozone, either alone or with other therapies.

Many of the well-known European health spas use ozone as a routine spa treatment for guests (a practice that may be compared with the regular tune-ups we give our cars), and a number of European physicians who treat patients with ozone also use it on themselves, even if they are not sick. These examples highlight the potential value of ozone and hydrogen peroxide as preventive therapies for cancer and many other diseases. An interesting project would be to study two groups of healthy people who may be genetically predisposed to cancer. One group could undergo bio-oxidative therapy for several years and any cases of cancer could be documented. The results could be enlightening and could form the basis for preventive cancer protocols for years to come.

6

HIV/AIDS

AIDS—acquired immunodeficiency syndrome—is perhaps the most feared disease on the planet. Usually fatal, it slowly destroys the immune system until the individual is vulnerable to a wide variety of diseases that rarely affect noninfected people. Those diseases may affect the brain, lungs, eyes, or other organs, like pneumocystis carinii pneumonia and Karposi sarcoma. People with AIDS also can experience debilitating weight loss, diarrhea, weakness, and depression.

AIDS is the most controversial disease of our time. Because it first affected primarily homosexuals, bisexuals, and intravenous drug users in the United States and other industrialized countries, critics of government health policy charged that society's negative feelings toward those groups led the government to be slow to respond to the growing epidemic. There is also a great deal of controversy surrounding the methods used to treat people with human immunodeficiency virus (HIV, the virus believed to cause AIDS) and AIDS.

AIDS has given birth to an entire "industry" involving physicians, nurses, hospitals, pharmaceutical companies, medical equipment manufacturers, government agencies, insurance companies, alternative therapists, testing laboratories, counselors, support groups, information networks, writers, publishers, researchers, educators, and magazines. Billions of dollars are involved in AIDS research, treatment, prevention, and education.

Physicians, scientists, and laypeople advocating the use of ozone and hydrogen peroxide can be included in this ever-expanding group.

Some are motivated by altruism and the desire to serve humanity, while others are primarily interested in money. For many providers of goods and services to AIDS patients, the epidemic has become an economic windfall of gigantic proportions. It is estimated that the United States Public Health Service's annual AIDS research budget was over $1.5 billion by 1994.[1] Burroughs Wellcome, the manufacturer of AZT, the most commonly used drug to stop replication of HIV, had sold $379 million worth of the drug during the 1992–1993 fiscal year.[2] For many physicians, hospitals, and insurance companies involved with AIDS, this disease is a big source of income and profit. For that reason, the quest to find inexpensive therapies and modalities to treat it is not a high priority.

A number of treatment protocols have been developed to combat the disease, based primarily on medications designed to stop the virus from replicating. Many new ones are being researched around the world. However, most approved medications have been only partially success-ful. Many patients do not respond to them, while others suffer adverse side effects, like anemia, pancreatitis, and neuropathy. And the long-term consequences of some of these medications are not yet known.

This has led people infected with the virus to explore other avenues of treatment, often using a combination of traditional and nontraditional approaches. These have included nontoxic therapies like acupuncture, acupressure, Chinese and Western herbs, ayurveda (an ancient Indian healing tradition that stresses diet and herbal medicines), homeopathy, chiropractic, and nutritional therapy.

Bio-oxidative therapies make up one of these approaches. The po-tential of ozone and hydrogen peroxide for helping people with HIV and AIDS is enormous, because laboratory evidence shows that ozone and hydrogen peroxide can inhibit (if not kill) the virus believed to cause AIDS. How does this happen?

Figure 6.1 depicts a chemical model of a virus that is about to infect a cell and shows how ozone can affect the process of infection. The virus is encapsulated in an envelope made of lipids (fats or fatlike sub-stances). Tiny bulbs on the virus spikes are known as receptors. It is through those receptors that a virus can connect with, and eventually infect, other cells. Through the application of ozone or hydrogen perox-ide (remember that when mixed with water, ozone becomes hydrogen peroxide), several events rapidly take place: The virus spikes are inactivated because the addition of ozone to the blood changes the

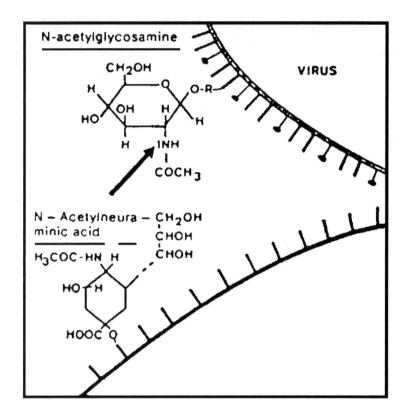

Figure 6.1. Chemical model of a virus and its encounter with ozone.
(From Siegfried Rilling and Renate Viebahn, The Use of Ozone in Medicine, *Heidelberg: Haug Publishers, 1987, 43. Reprinted courtesy of Dr. Siegfried Rilling and Haug Publishers.)*

structure of the receptor. Although still alive, the virus cannot join with the cell. At the same time, the ozone oxidates the virus's outer envelope. Without that envelope, it cannot survive.

In addition to the effects of hydrogen peroxide introduced from outside the body, the threatened cell naturally defends itself by producing its own hydrogen peroxide. In some cases, especially when a cell is unhealthy to begin with, the hydrogen peroxide it produces causes it to "burst" before reproduction of the virus can take place. In other cases, the peroxides introduced by added ozone or hydrogen peroxide act synergistically with the hydrogen peroxide inside a cell, destroying any virus that has penetrated it.[3] Stated more simply: If the cell is unhealthy to begin with, it is destroyed by a hydrogen peroxide burst. If it is strong, it kills off the virus and becomes even stronger due to the increased oxygenation. As a result, the virus is either inactivated or destroyed.

Another possible benefit of ozone therapy for people with HIV is its ability to stimulate the production of superoxide dismutase, a vital enzyme that catalyzes the conversion of two molecules of superoxide into one molecule of oxygen and one molecule of hydrogen peroxide. According to a report in *American Medical News*, researchers at the Webb–Waring Institute in Denver discovered that HIV inhibits the body's natural production of superoxide dismutase. The news release added that researchers are testing human cell cultures to elucidate if a drug can inhibit HIV's ability to suppress the enzyme. They believe that if they are able to safeguard the enzyme's levels in cells, the time HIV stays inactive could be prolonged. This finding points to the value of ozone therapy in helping prevent HIV-related symptoms from manifesting.[4]

As powerful immunomodulators, ozone and hydrogen peroxide can also strengthen a compromised immune system. They can help guard against opportunistic infections and enable people suffering from the disease to lead longer, more active, and more productive lives. While bio-oxidative therapies should not be considered a cure for AIDS, they may open the door to long-term remission, especially when used in synergistic combination with other immune-strengthening therapies. Investigations are now proceeding to delineate such combinations, including ozone and/or hydrogen peroxide and oral alpha interferon, staph vaccine, lentinan (shiitake mushroom extract), and Chinese herbs. Readers interested in updates regarding these combinations may contact an organization called Keep Hope Alive (see North American Organizations in the resources section).

First, Some Background

According to the United States Centers for Disease Control and Prevention, HIV disease is characterized by a gradual deterioration of immune function. During the course of the disease, specific body cells (called CD4 +T-cells) are disabled and killed. Those cells, which are also called T-helper cells, are white blood cells that orchestrate the body's immune response and signal other cells in the immune system to perform their functions. Other immune cells with CD4 molecules (such as macrophage) are infected as well.

Healthy people usually have between 800 and 1200 CD4+T-cells (also known as CD4 cells) per microliter of blood. When the number of T-helper cells falls below 200 cells per microliter, a person can become vulnerable to a variety of life-threatening opportunistic infections and cancers, including pneumocystis carinii pneumonia (PCP), Karposi sarcoma, toxoplasmosis, meningitis, and one or more classes of lymphoma. Individuals who have been shown to be infected with HIV are officially diagnosed with AIDS when their T-helper cell count is under 400 and they come down with one or more opportunistic infections (especially PCP) or if their T-helper cell count falls below 200, even if they are asymptomatic.[5]

The World Health Organization (WHO) estimates that since the beginning of the HIV/AIDS epidemic, approximately 11.7 million people around the world died from AIDS by mid-1997 out of approximately 30.6 million who were infected with HIV. It estimated that 860,000 adults and children were living with HIV/AIDS in North America alone.[6]

The human immunodeficiency virus was first isolated in the laboratory in 1983 and was determined to be the cause of AIDS the following year, because it was found to be present in the blood of people suffering from the disease. Since HIV is found in blood, semen, and other body fluids, scientists established that the major avenues of transmission included sexual intercourse, the sharing of needles among drug users, and HIV-infected blood transfusions.

Given the enormous threat of this disease, a number of drug companies devoted their efforts to developing expensive medications that could stop the replication of the virus, if not kill it completely. Attention became centered on the process of *reverse transcription*, in which the virus's unique enzyme (known as reverse transcriptase) converts the single-stranded RNA into DNA after the virus has entered a cell. That is what makes the virus multiply and why it is classified as a *retrovirus*. As of this writing, the three approved drugs developed for that purpose in the United States are zidovudine, or azidothymidine (AZT), dianosine (ddl), and zalcitabine (ddC). All three are controversial. A number of clinical studies have disputed their effectiveness. The drugs are very expensive, and all can produce adverse side effects.

It is important to remember that the presence of HIV does not mean that the individual will invariably come down with AIDS. When AIDS first became a public health issue in the early 1980s, authorities declared that infected people would develop AIDS within eighteen months to three years. That time frame has now increased to an average of ten years or longer. In addition, the blood test for HIV does not measure the amount of virus in the blood: When a person is tested positive for HIV, it means that that person's immune system has produced antibodies to counteract the virus. While this may well indicate that the person is vulnerable to the replication of the virus, it also can mean that the person's immune system has been able to fight the virus off.

Although few people disagree that AIDS destroys the body's immune system, a growing number of researchers, physicians, and patients have taken issue with the "one cause" theory for AIDS and the established approaches for treatment. This is important in our discussion, because bio-oxidative therapies act against the disease in a number of different ways. Perhaps the best-known critic is Dr. Peter Duisberg, a professor of molecular biology at the University of California at Berkeley. Considered the foremost authority on retroviruses, he refuted the original HIV/AIDS hypothesis in the *Proceedings of the New York Academy of Sciences* in 1989.[7]

At a landmark conference in Amsterdam in May 1992, Dr. Duisberg joined several hundred scientists, physicians, alternative health practitioners, AIDS activists, and patients (including long-term survivors) to discuss the definition and politics of AIDS, how HIV infects the body, and how the disease can be treated through alternative means. According to a report on the conference in the consumer letter *Health Facts*, the causative factors most considered were these:

> Sexually transmitted diseases and their treatments; intravenous and recreational drug use, particularly "poppers," which are nitrite inhalants used to enhance orgasms and numb the pain of repeated violent sex for the passive partner; chronic use of high-dose antibiotics and other prescription drugs; contamination from blood transfusions; and multiple viral and bacterial diseases (e.g., hepatitis, parasites).[8]

Attention was focused on the possibility that the person is *already* immunosuppressed and that the HIV virus, if it is a factor at all, is only taking advantage of a previously compromised immune system rather than being the cause of it. Others, such as Michael Ellner from the New York alternative AIDS organization HEAL (Health Education AIDS Liaison), regard "AIDS as a condition of toxicity rather than a viral disease; it is a disturbance of immune function caused by a lifetime of toxins."[9]

This view was also proposed to me during a recent interview with Dr. Juliane Sacher of Frankfurt, who has one of the largest medical practices treating AIDS patients with ozone in Germany. She placed special emphasis on the combined effects of air pollution (especially in the large cities), the growing number of pesticides in our food supply, the widespread use of antibiotics and other immune-suppressing drugs, recreational drug use, eating heavily processed and devitalized foods, and a variety of vitamin and mineral deficiencies that occur as a result. For this reason, she believes that a greater emphasis should be placed on building up the person's immune system while assisting the patient to become (and remain) as free of toxins as possible.[10]

Although I cite the laboratory evidence that ozone can inactivate the human immunodeficiency virus (and that some people who once tested HIV-positive reverted to HIV-negative), I reiterate that neither ozone nor hydrogen peroxide is a cure for AIDS. However, if correctly applied, they can play an important role in a holistic approach to treatment. This perspective was succinctly expressed in a communication from Frank Shallenberger, M.D., H.M.D., of Nevada, who has treated HIV patients with ozone and other natural therapies:

1. Ozone therapy does *not* cure AIDS—[it] never has and probably never will.

2. AIDS has a multi-faceted causation and is *not* an infectious disease. Therapy for AIDS will *never* work if it is only aimed at anti-infectious protocol.

3. Ozone therapy works in AIDS by acting as an immune system modulator. In this capacity, it is very effective, safe, inexpensive, and readily available.

4. Proper therapy for AIDS will be directed at

   • early intervention (i.e., CD4 count >300)

   • ozone plus other synergistic immune-augmented therapy

   • intestinal cleansing is paramount due to the immunosuppressive aspect of parasites.[11]

The following pages will explore the laboratory and clinical findings related to HIV, plus the ways that ozone and hydrogen peroxide are being used by patients today.

In Vitro Studies

In vitro studies to evaluate the ability of ozone to kill the human immuno-deficiency virus in the test tube have been undertaken by eminent scientists in the United States, Russia, and Canada.

The first researchers in the world to prove that ozone can inactivate the human immunodeficiency virus were Michael T. F. Carpendale, M.D. (chief of medicine and research services at the Veterans Administration Hospital in San Francisco and professor at the University of California School of Medicine, San Francisco), and his associate, Dr. Joel K. Freeberg of the Veterans Administration Hospital. They first presented their findings at the Fourth International Conference of AIDS in Stockholm in 1988 and later published their report in the peer-reviewed journal *Antiviral Research*. Carpendale and Freeberg showed that HIV could be 99 percent inactivated with only 0.5 µg ozone/ml of human serum, and completely inactivated by ozone concentrations of 4 µg/ml of human serum. Those concentrations of ozone did not harm healthy cells.[12]

Another in vitro study, supported in part by the U.S. Public Health Service and Medizone International, a manufacturer of a patented medical ozone delivery system, was reported in the October 1, 1991, issue of the medical journal *Blood*. Using ozone generated from medical-grade oxygen and delivered into a cultured cell medium of HIV-1, a team of four scientists from the SUNY Health Science Center in Syracuse, the Brooklyn Hospital, and Merck Pharmaceutical found that ozone deactivated the virus completely without causing significant biological damage to noninfected cells. In evaluating their findings with HIV, the researchers concluded:

> The data indicate that the antiviral effects of ozone include viral particle disruption, reverse transcriptase inactivation, and/or a perturbation of the ability of the virus to bind its receptor to target cells.[13]

In Russia, scientists at the Institute of Virusology in Moscow also used a concentration of 4 µg/ml of ozone on an infected culture containing the human immunodeficiency virus. Within minutes, the cell of the virus decomposed and died. The researchers noted that "complete deactivation of [the] extra cell virus is achieved by putting gaseous ozone through [the] virus-containing [liquid]."[14]

In chapter 2, brief reference was made to a major study in Canada, which was coordinated by the surgeon general of the Canadian Armed Forces, to determine the ability of ozone to kill HIV, hepatitis, and herpes viruses in blood used for transfusion. After a three-minute ozonation of serum spiked with one million HIV-1 particles per milliliter, a 100 percent deactivation of the virus was achieved.[15] Referring to this study during his interview in the video documentary "Ozone and the Politics of Medicine," Captain Michael E. Shannon, a scientist and medical doctor with the Canadian Department of National Defence, said: "We are dealing not with concentrations that are toxic to the human, but (are in fact) concentrations of ozone that have been used in clinics in Germany for the last thirty years with thousands of patients without any evidence of any harm."[16]

Despite the importance of the results (which indicate that ozonation of the blood supply would render it free of HIV, as well as herpes, hepatitis, and other viruses), the Canadian findings received little notice in the mainstream North American press.

Clinical Experience

Germany

Dr. Horst Kief, who is perhaps best known for his work with patients suffering from cancer and neurodermatitis, as well as the development of AHIT, is believed to be the first physician in the world to treat AIDS patients with hyperbaric ozone "blood washings," in the early 1980s. His standard protocol has consisted of a session of autohemotherapy once a week for three months, which can be repeated if necessary.

In a monograph published in the German medical journal *Erfahrungheilkunde* in July 1988, Dr. Kief wrote that the early patients experienced a near-complete alleviation of various AIDS-related symptoms, including thrush and oral hairy leukoplakia. In addition, their T4-cell counts increased dramatically as well as the T4:T8 ratio over a time period of sixty-five days.[17] In an interview shown in "Ozone and the Politics of Medicine," Dr. Kief said that a seven-year follow-up of his first patients found them alive, working, and "doing very, very well."[18]

However, the first documented cases of using ozone to treat AIDS were published by the German physician Alexander Pruess in 1986. In his work with four patients, Dr. Pruess used ozone in combination with

Suramin (a reverse transcriptase inhibitor), immunomodulation therapy, vitamin and mineral supplementation, and the hygienation of intestinal flora (bacteria present in the intestines). He decided to use ozone because

> As it is well-known that the actual disease(s) occurring through AIDS consists of a combination of viral, fungal and bacteriological infections, I searched for a substance which is viricidal, fungicidal and bactericidal at the same time. Ozone was here the obvious choice. . . .[19]

Dr. Pruess noted immediate improvement in all four patients, including the elimination of HIV-related problems like skin diseases, fungal infections, gastrointestinal problems, and low energy. Over a year after treatment, all subjects were considered clinically healthy.

In a monograph published in 1993, Dr. Kief wrote about a study comparing thirty patients from the Kief Clinic who were given ozone in the form of AHIT and twenty patients from the University of Frankfurt School of Medicine who received conventional treatment, including AZT. Dr. Kief's patients were observed over 251 days, while the Frankfurt patients were observed for 363 days. T4:T8 ratios rose from 0.324 to 0.352 among Kief's patients, whereas they fell from 0.293 to 0.223 among the Frankfurt patients.

In a related study of twenty-seven AIDS patients receiving AHIT, the percentage surviving after eighteen months was 80 percent, and the percentage surviving after forty-five months was 70 percent. This represents a much higher percentage than patients receiving conventional medical therapy anywhere.[20]

While these figures are encouraging, Dr. Kief is no longer using AHIT to treat people with AIDS. In 1992, German health authorities ordered him to create and maintain a separate (and highly secure) laboratory to make AHIT for his HIV and AIDS patients. Since the cost to build and secure a new facility was prohibitively expensive, Dr. Kief decided to stop using AHIT, and his HIV/AIDS practice is presently confined to treating patients with major autohemotherapy.

United States

In the United States, pilot studies were developed in the late 1980s by Dr. Michael T. Carpendale and Dr. John Griffiss of the Department of Laboratory Medicine at the University of California School of Medicine in San Francisco to find out if there is a role for medical ozone in the treatment of HIV and associated infections.

In a study using two asymptomatic people infected with HIV, one (known as Patient G) began with a T-cell count of 309, while the other (Patient I) began with a T-cell count of 907. The treatment protocol consisted of doses of ozone and oxygen given via rectal insufflation daily for twenty-one days, once every three days for sixteen weeks, and once weekly for fifteen weeks, for a total of seventy-three treatments over a period of thirty-four weeks. For the next two years, the subjects treated themselves with a three-week "booster dose," which was repeated from time to time, as seen in figure 6.2.

The researchers reported that T-cell levels remained acceptable (i.e., over 430) over the next six years, and both individuals "remained in the best of health, with increased feeling of well being and energy, while on ozone therapy and with no infections and no adverse symptoms of malaise for the first five years." By that time, Patient I, who began the study with a higher T-cell level, had not only attained a T-cell count of 1185 but also tested HIV-negative. Three months into the sixth year, however, Patient G died suddenly from lobar pneumonia (not AIDS-related PCP pneumonia) after getting soaked in a storm while recuperating from the flu. When he died, Patient G was still HIV-positive, yet he had maintained a T-cell count between 500 and 700.

In their report, which was published in *Ozone in Medicine: Proceedings of the Eleventh Ozone World Congress,* the researchers concluded:

> These normalizing results support the hypothesis that ozone may be effective in suppressing and possibly eliminating HIV, especially in the stages of the disease when the patient is asymptomatic and has a CD4 cell count in the normal range. It also indicates the potential for self treatment for long term prophylaxis, treatment or care.[21]

In a related study, which was published in the *Journal of Clinical Gastroenterology,* Dr. Carpendale and his associates treated five AIDS patients suffering from intractable diarrhea with daily colonic insufflations of ozone (at doses from 2.7 to 30 mg) for twenty-one to twenty-eight days. By the end of the study, three of the four patients were completely relieved of their symptoms, while one patient, whose diarrhea was the result of the parasite cryptosporidium, experienced no change. Relief from secondary infections, including herpes simplex, folliculitis, and sycosis barbae, was also reported. Patients

Figure 6.2. Absolute CD4 ("T") cell count in HIV+ patients treated with ozone plotted against time. (From Michael T. Carpendale, M.D., and John Griffiss, M.D., "Is There a Role for Medical Ozone in the Treatment of HIV and Associated Infections?" in Ozone in Medicine: Proceedings of the Eleventh Ozone World Congress, Stamford, Conn., International Ozone Association, Pan American Committee, 1993, M–1–39, 40.)

experienced less toxicity, less discomfort, and more energy than before being treated with ozone. No adverse side effects were reported.[22]

Dr. Carpendale was so encouraged by the results of these studies that he has attempted to secure government funding for additional ozone studies involving many more people. He has met with no success so far.

The results of another pilot study with ozone were presented at the Fourth International Bio-Oxidative Medicine Conference in April 1993 by Dr. Frank Shallenberger. Considered one of the leading authorities on medical ozone in the United States, Dr. Shallenberger administered intravenous ozone over a period of fourteen days, to five randomly selected men diagnosed with AIDS. The total daily dose was calculated to be 0.15 µg ozone/kg body weight. On the first day, one-fourth the daily dose was given, on the second, one-half, and the third, three-fourths. From the fourth to the fourteenth day, the full dose was administered. Patients were carefully monitored and evaluated before and after each treatment. During the period after therapy, no other therapies were given, except in the case of one patient, who began taking ddI after the fourth month.

Before the ozone treatments began, each patient participated in a holistic protocol including a whole-foods nutritional program, meditation and deep breathing, lymphatic drainage massage, nutritional supplements, safe sex practices, and regular exercise.

Although Dr. Shallenberger considered the sample too small to be statistically significant, the results included at least a six-month period of overall survival, an immediate increase in the number of T-cells, relief of symptoms from opportunistic infections among most patients, and higher energy levels overall. Dr. Shallenberger's clinical observations follow:

1. S.W. (34 years old): Diffuse cutaneous Karposi Sarcoma of two year duration went into clinical remission for six months before the lesions returned. Otherwise continues to be in good health.

2. S.S. (27 years old): Chronic diarrhea (cryptosporidium), chronic fatigue, and weight loss >20%. All symptoms disappeared within two months, and the patient remains healthy one year later. CD4 count remains at 7.

3. R.J. (34 years old): Oral thrush, fatigue, and mild lymphadenopathy [swollen lymph nodes]. Thrush disappeared for six months. Fatigue is gone. Lymphadenopathy has not progressed, and the patient remains in good health one year later.

4. T.B. (32 years old): Hairy leukoplakia and mild lymphadenopathy. Neither of these symptoms changed. He remains in otherwise good health one year later.

5. M.P. (41 years old): Neuro-leukodystrophy. Needs assistance to walk, has urinary incontinence and impotence. Within one week of treatment his incontinence and gait improved considerably. One month later, he was walking easily without assistance and had no incontinence. MRI remains stable, showing no progression of lesions, as does the patient at a ten-month interval.[23]

Dr. Shallenberger's findings support the hypothesis that ozone therapy can have long-term positive effects on AIDS patients. While not a cure, ozone therapy can play a role in improving the quality of life of people living with AIDS.

Positive results from bio-oxidative therapies were also reported by John C. Pittman, M.D., of North Carolina. Having worked extensively with HIV and AIDS patients over several years, his holistic treatments including ozone and hydrogen peroxide helped a number of patients to become HIV-negative. He also began to collect data relating to HIV-infected patients who received bio-oxidative therapy throughout the country.

One of those patients was a thirty-four-year-old man referred to as D.M. who was diagnosed HIV-positive in March 1991 and had a CD4+ T-cell count of 600, considered to be in the low range of normal. In April 1991 he began receiving autohemotherapy once a day for ten days, along with intravenous hydrogen peroxide and intravenous vitamins, including especially large amounts of vitamin C. In July, he repeated a thirty-day treatment protocol with ozone, hydrogen peroxide, vitamins, and antiviral compounds, as well as nutritional therapies designed to aid in intestinal cleansing and metabolic detoxification. During the first two weeks of therapy, D. M. experienced fever and a drop in his T-cell count to 400, which Dr. Pittman attributed to a die-off of virus particles and infected lymphocytes. Following the thirty-day protocol, D. M. reported that his enlarged neck and inguinal lymph nodes became much smaller. Laboratory tests showed that his CD4+ T-cell count rose to 900.

D. M. continued receiving occasional treatments with ozone and vitamin C and by November 1992, his T-helper cell count had reached 1400, and his enlarged lymph nodes had returned to normal. Although D. M. still tested HIV-positive, there was no sign of viral activity by P24 antigen testing.[24] An antigen is a substance that induces the formation of antibodies.

After Dr. Pittman was ordered to stop using bio-oxidative therapies or have his practice closed by state medical authorities in 1993, he decided to set up an AIDS clinic in Haiti. After North Carolina passed the Alternative Medical Practices Act in 1994, Dr. Pittman was advised that he could return to North Carolina, where he now practices ozone therapy on an experimental basis.

Like Dr. Shallenberger's, Dr. Pittman's treatment protocol encompasses a holistic approach. He recommends using intravenous ozone, intravenous hydrogen peroxide, intravenous vitamin C, EDTA chelation (involving the intravenous administration of EDTA, a synthetic amino acid), external oxygenation (baths with ozone and hydrogen peroxide), hyperbaric oxygen, metabolic and intestinal detoxification, a raw and living food diet, nutritional supplements, and exercise.[25] Dr. Pittman's protocol is examined in more detail later on. His nonprofit organization Cure AIDS Now (see resources) is devoted to collecting evidence of successful treatment of HIV infection with bio-oxidative therapies.

Canada

Heartened by the in vitro blood studies by the Canadian armed forces, the government decided to sponsor a study with actual AIDS patients. Coordinated by Captain Michael E. Shannon, M.D., in collaboration with Dr. Michael O'Shaughnessy, a virologist with the Laboratory Centre for Disease Control in Ottawa, the study employed twenty-four volunteers suffering from AIDS in two trials using minor autohemotherapy. The Phase I study, which involved ten patients, showed an increase of T-cells among those who had 300 or more to begin with, while those who had 90 T-cells or less experienced a decrease.[26] A Phase II random study was then begun with fourteen patients, half to receive ozone treatments and half a placebo. The findings were inconclusive, however, because the ozone generator used in the study failed to produce ozone. Since the study was double blinded, no one knew about the defect until it was too late.

However, in a personal communication I received from Captain Shannon in January 1994, he wrote:

> Of interest, however, the three patients (out of ten volunteers) who responded to minor autohemotherapy in the *first trial*, are still alive after four years post-treatment, with CD4 counts in excess of two hundred. These patients theoretically should have succumbed to AIDS within a year post-treatment.[27]

Captain Shannon added that although those initial results must still be explained, there was little interest within the Health Protection Branch of Health and Welfare Canada to pursue the matter further.

In a letter dated January 13, 1995, addressed to Ed McCabe, Dr. Shannon (who by that time had been promoted to the rank of Commander and appointed Deputy Surgeon General of Canada) offered his candid evaluation of the future of ozone in treating patients with HIV and contradicted the views of one of the other researchers who participated in the second study. At Dr. Shannon's request, the letter is reproduced in its entirety.

> Notwithstanding the negative findings of Dr. Garber's 1991 clinical trial, I firmly believe that ozone therapy has potential to play a valuable role in the medical management of AIDS. From a regulatory point of view, it is clear that not all forms of ozone therapy will be considered sufficiently safe and/or efficacious in this regard; however, there is no doubt in my mind that a protocol will eventually emerge with proven benefit.
>
> Looking back at my past experience with minor autohemotherapy in the treatment of AIDS, there still remains a discrepancy between the Phase 1a and 1b trial results, which may, in part, relate to the lack of sophisticated technology to control for O_3 concentrations in both trials. Given the lack of any significant therapeutic breakthroughs in the treatment of AIDS since that ill-fated trial and the growing testimonial support for its efficacy, the need for further clinical research with ozone is certainly indicated. It is indeed unfortunate that the North American medical community and its funding agencies could not take a more neutral stance on this subject; tragically, professional opinion has been somewhat polarized on this issue. I believe that it is time to take the emotion out of the arguments, both pro and con, and commence a systematic examination of the evidence currently available on the merits of this therapy. Where information gaps exist (particularly in peer-reviewed scientific studies) which might preclude any regulatory decision on the validity of certain claims, properly designed research initiatives should be encouraged with the same kind of public support normally afforded any other scientific endeavour of this import.[28]

At the time of this writing, no large-scale research is being done on the ability of ozone to treat AIDS. Medizone International, which holds a patent on a unique medical ozone delivery system, is engaged in a multicentered Phase II clinical trial in Italy using major autohemotherapy, while two smaller studies are being sponsored by independent research foundations in the United States.

Cuba

AIDS is not a major health problem in Cuba. When the AIDS epidemic first came to light, everyone on the island was tested for HIV infection, and the several hundred who tested positive (many of whom are believed to have contracted the virus in Angola, where Cuba was involved in military operations) were quarantined by the government. They were placed in campuslike settings and given free housing, medical care, and healthy food but were not allowed to leave the area. This policy has recently been liberalized for those who are not likely to spread the virus to the general population.

During my interviews with scientists from the National Center for Scientific Research in Havana, I learned that ozone had been given to several of the detainees with some success, although undertaking a study of ozone to treat AIDS is not a high priority due to the low number of infected people.

Dr. Silvia Menéndez, a chemist who cofounded the Centro de Ozono with Dr. Manuel Gómez in 1985, told me that ozone works best when administered as soon as possible after infection, before the virus has penetrated the lymphatic system and bone marrow. She believed that, If caught early, ozone could deactivate the virus in the blood and prevent it from infecting other cells. She added that ozone therapy could help prevent and treat some of the opportunistic infections that are common among AIDS patients.[29]

Her comment regarding the early use of ozone for those infected with HIV is very important. If a person could be treated with ozone *as soon as possible after infection*, perhaps the normal progression of the disease could be interrupted. The economic and social ramifications of this possibility cannot be underestimated.

Anecdotal Findings

Over the years, hundreds of anecdotal reports regarding the positive results of bio-oxidative therapies for the treatment of HIV infection and AIDS have surfaced. Many of those reports come from patients and their physicians, many of whom must remain anonymous. The use of medical ozone generators is illegal in most states and Canadian provinces, and physicians who use them—if discovered—can lose their medical licenses or be put in jail.

J. P. of Milwaukee was first diagnosed HIV-positive in 1988 and had a T-cell count of 237 in June 1992. He decided to use Viroterm (a type of oral alpha interferon) and ozone through the sauna-bag method over a period of several months. After three weeks of using ozone daily, J. P. found that his lymph nodes, which had been swollen for three years, subsided to normal. In addition, his T-cell counts increased from 237 (in June) to 292 (in October). In June, he had tested positive for P24, a protein found in the core of the human immunodeficiency virus, and by October, his doctor told him that he had tested negative for P24.[30] Further details on the use of the sauna-bag method by HIV/AIDS patients can be found in the sixth edition of *AIDS Control Diet* and in *HIV Treatment News,* published by Keep Hope Alive (see resources).

Brad J. is a registered nurse who was stuck with a needle while taking blood from an AIDS patient in June 1991. By November he tested positive for HIV, as well as hepatitis B and C. His T-cells dropped substantially, and by February he had lost thirty pounds, was extremely fatigued, and suffered from severe diarrhea, making it almost impossible to work. Despite his physician's advice, he refused to take AZT and began intravenous infusions of vitamin C five times a week, which caused the diarrhea to abate from twenty movements a day to six. In December 1992, he met Ed McCabe, who told him about ozone, and the following February Brad traveled to Germany to become a certified practitioner in ozone therapy. However, it was not until April 1993 that Brad began taking ozone via autohemotherapy himself every seventy-two hours for three months. By the second treatment the diarrhea was eliminated, and he felt his old energy return. His hepatitis symptoms disappeared, and his viral load index became undetectable.

Brad has continued using ozone sporadically over the past four years, augmented with Chinese herbs and vitamin C. Since he finds autohemotherapy uncomfortable, Brad currently administers ozone in each ear once or twice a week. His health situation is stable: After four years, he has been free of HIV-related symptoms and his T-cells remain at about 400. In addition to his full time job as a nurse, Brad maintains a practice as a biofeedback therapist; he has also been assisting physicians set up ozone clinics. Although Brad credits his good health partly to a spiritual awakening and the use of vitamins and herbs, he says bluntly, "Ozone saved my life."

Another man (whom we will call Bill) was tested HIV-positive in early 1982 and by 1993 had a T-cell count of 36. In August of that year, he began using the sauna-bag method and reported that his breathing difficulties disappeared after three treatments. He also experienced relief of a chronic herpes problem. He began rectal insufflation with humidified ozone in November twice a day and reported relief of abdominal pain and an improved ability to sleep.

Although the exact dose of ozone to be given via rectal insufflation for each individual patient should be determined by a physician, Michael Carpendale, M.D., disclosed the protocol he used in his San Francisco clinical investigations with AIDS patients at the Eleventh Ozone World Congress in 1993:

> Ozone was produced from a portable medical ozone generator (Hansler, Iffezheim, Germany), and was insufflated through a teflon catheter into the colon. This is a simple, safe, inexpensive and well documented method for treatment with ozone. Dosage concentration was 22–30 mg O_3/ml O_2; average volume was 1100 ml for a total dose of 26.2–33 mg O_3 per treatment. The treatment program was daily for twenty-one days, once every three days for sixteen weeks, and once weekly for fifteen weeks, for a total of thirty-four to thirty-six weeks and seventy-three treatments containing 2065–2137 mg ozone.[31]

Further information regarding the rectal insufflation method to treat HIV/AIDS can be found in the literature published by Keep Hope Alive.

John from Illinois had a T-cell count in the 200 range and began taking five drops of 35 percent food-grade hydrogen peroxide in water three times a day about three hours after meals. He gradually increased the dose to twenty drops, which he maintained for two months. He then reduced it to five drops and got tested again. His T-cell count had risen to 800. In his comments on the case, Mark Konlee, the author of *AIDS Control Diet*, did not recommend using oral hydrogen peroxide; he added that the same results could be obtained by adding a pint of food-grade hydrogen peroxide to warm bath water and soaking in it for twenty minutes a day.[32]

AIDS and the Politics of Bio-oxidative Therapies

The use of bio-oxidative therapies is fraught with controversy. The pharmaceutical companies—which stand to make billions of dollars in profits from anti-AIDS medications—are completely opposed to the use of cheap, safe, and potentially effective substances like hydrogen peroxide and ozone in treating this disease. In addition, many physicians are either ignorant of or hostile toward therapies that can be self-administered, like the sauna-bag and rectal-insufflation methods mentioned.

Many reputable and caring physicians who have treated AIDS patients with ozone and hydrogen peroxide have been threatened by state licensing authorities and have had their practices closed down. The United States Food and Drug Administration and the National Institutes of Health have refused to sponsor human trials for ozone and hydrogen peroxide and have made it extremely difficult for small independent companies like Medizone International to undertake such research. Despite the fact that over ten million people (including over a thousand AIDS patients) have received ozone therapy in Europe and that reliable data on the use of ozone and hydrogen peroxide are supported by hundreds of scientific articles and clinical studies, the FDA maintains that bio-oxidative therapies like ozone have not been proven either safe or effective. In the words of Dr. Randolph F. Wykoff, the director of the Office of AIDS Coordination and the acting associate commissioner for Science, Food and Drug Administration, testifying before the Committee on the Judiciary Subcommittee on Crime and Criminal Justice at the House of Representatives in Washington on May 27, 1993:

> Ozone therapy has also been used to treat AIDS patients without any scientific data to support the agent's safety or effectiveness. Ozone therapy and ozone generators have been promoted in magazines and newspaper advertisements and in books, videos, and audio cassettes. The introduction of ozone into immunosuppressed AIDS patients without careful study of probable toxicities places the patients at unreasonable and significant risks.[33]

The political and economic situation in the United States and Canada has led many patients to seek treatment elsewhere, primarily in Mexico. While there are several reputable clinics in this country, some unethical promoters have held out promises for a cure at a price approaching

$20,000. One scheme even offered patients six-figure salaries if they would promote their success to other prospective patients later on, especially to those who owned homes that could be mortgaged for $100,000 to pay for treatment.[34]

Until health-care consumers speak out to their elected representatives, we will continue to be denied the right to choose the forms of health care we want. Large-scale clinical studies regarding the effectiveness of ozone and hydrogen peroxide to treat AIDS will never be done, and funding for research will continue to fall on the individual researchers themselves. Doctors will be forced to continue administering these therapies illegally and surreptitiously, and many people without access to those physicians will continue to self-administer ozone or hydrogen peroxide. While amazingly few adverse side effects have been reported, no one should ever be forced to self-medicate without the benefit of supervision from a qualified health professional. Entrepreneurs eager to fill their pockets will offer magical cures costing tens of thousands of dollars, while many individuals who are infected with HIV or who are dying of AIDS will decide to "go for broke" and try untested treatments from clinics of dubious reputation. Those with the strength and the financial resources may choose to leave their families and friends and seek reliable care in Germany or Cuba.

7

ADDITIONAL APPLICATIONS OF BIO-OXIDATIVE THERAPIES

In addition to heart disease, cancer, and HIV infection, the scope of health problems that have responded to bio-oxidative therapies is very broad. In the following pages, we examine the clinical and laboratory evidence gathered from reputable medical and scientific sources from around the world. As with the earlier presentations, readers are invited to consult the original references listed in the notes section.

Allergies

Each year over a hundred patients with allergies go to the Kief Clinic in Ludwigshafen, Germany, for ozone and autohomologous immunotherapy (AHIT). Many of them have not responded to conventional medical treatment, including antibiotics and steroids, and visit the clinic as a last resort.

In a statistical analysis of thirty-nine patients treated with AHIT, one-third experienced a full remission of symptoms, 22 percent had significant improvement, and one-third showed some improvement. Eleven percent did not respond to AHIT.[1]

Analgesic Properties

In the AIDS trials undertaken by the Canadian Department of Defence in 1990, the analgesic effects of ozone were discovered unexpectedly. According to Captain Michael Shannon, M.D., who coordinated the study, "Inadvertently, we discovered that this particular type of therapy has an incredible effect, a very pronounced effect in managing pain. It has a very potent analgesic effect."[2]

I personally observed the analgesic effects of intravenous hydrogen peroxide on an individual who was suffering from a variety of serious AIDS-related symptoms and was given only a few weeks to live. Daily intravenous hydrogen peroxide given at home appeared to relieve much of his discomfort, lift his spirits, facilitate sleep, and increase his overall energy level. Although the patient died, the quality of his final days was dramatically improved.

Arthrosis

Arthrosis is a disease that involves the progressive degeneration of cartilage in the spine, knees, and other joints. Like arthritis, arthrosis causes intense pain and limits movement. In 1990, Cuban researchers studied 230 patients complaining of pain and related problems in the lumbosacral spine, knee, and other joints. A total of twenty intramuscular injections of oxygen and ozone were given over a period of twenty days, one injection daily for the first ten days and one injection every other day for an additional twenty days. All patients were carefully examined, diagnosed, and evaluated before the study.

The results were impressive: 208 patients (89 percent) reported complete disappearance of pain, 24 (10 percent) reported some degree of relief; only two patients (1 percent) reported no change in their health status. In follow-up examinations, the researchers found that most of the patients remained symptom free from three to six months, while some did not feel pain for up to eleven months after treatment. People with herniated spinal discs also felt relief with ozone therapy.[3]

Due to improved treatment methods, those results were even better than an earlier Cuban study of 122 arthrosis patients, in which 71.8 percent of the patients treated with ozone reported complete relief of pain, while 21.8 percent reported improvement.[4]

A 1988 study undertaken by Dr. E. Riva Sanseverino at the University of Bologna in Italy focused on the effects of injected oxygen and ozone on different types of knee disorders, primarily arthrosis of the knee joint. On hundred fifty-six patients were divided into three groups depending on symptoms: Group A (forty-four patients) suffered from post-traumatic knee disorders, Group B (83 patients) were diagnosed with gonarthrosis (arthrosis of the knee joint) without bone deformity, and Group C (29 patients) had gonarthrosis with bone deformity. Ten patients (7 from Group B and 3 from Group C) had both knees treated, but one knee was treated with oxygen alone.

Patients in Group A were given two to four injections a week for six weeks, while members of the other groups were treated with three cycles of oxygen–ozone injections over a period of fourteen months. In evaluating the effects of treatment, attention was given to improved flexion–extension mobility of the knee, pain reduction, and reduction in swelling.

The results showed that only ozone-treated knees showed improvement. Overall, Dr. Riva Sanseverino concluded that

> oxygen–ozone therapy is extremely efficient in cases of acute knee traumata (Group A) and in all those forms of knee disorders where the degenerative process is at the beginning (Group B). In these two conditions, a prediction is possible for total or almost total recovery.

The patients in Group C, whose knee degeneration was more advanced, required additional medical therapies on a prolonged basis.

At the conclusion of his article, Dr. Riva Sanseverino stressed the high degree of safety of low doses of medical ozone and the absence of adverse side effects: "The absolute absence of any negative collateral effect of the local ozone treatment deserves great consideration."[5]

Bronchial Asthma

Very few studies of patients suffering from bronchial asthma have been undertaken. However, during a research visit to Cuba, I was introduced to an eleven-year-old boy at a special school for the hearing-impaired whose asthma was cured with ozone. Ricardo was originally treated for hypocusia, a disease of the inner ear that causes deafness. The ozone treatments he received provided a modest degree of hearing improvement, which was consistent with the results of the other students of the school who were given ozone for hypocusia. However, along with improved hearing, Ricardo's parents and teachers noticed that his frequent asthma attacks gradually began to diminish and then to nearly disappear.

Dr. Gilbert Glady, a French physician, reported his clinical experience with an asthma patient at the Eleventh Ozone World Congress that was held in San Francisco in 1993. (The English in his written report has been corrected where necessary.)

> Mrs. Nicole B., born in 1947, had been suffering from bronchial asthma since 1981. She was treated with Lomudal and Aminophylline as well as with antibiotics every time she was suffering from ear, nose or throat infections. The tests showed an allergy to house dusts. We met her for the first time in December 1987 at a period when she had attacks of asthma nearly every day. An ozone treatment involving alternate doses of minor autohemotherapy in the form of subcutaneous injections at the top of the lungs and major autohemotherapy was started in February 1988. . . .
>
> After about ten sessions, the frequency of attacks of asthma had decreased substantially, although some secondary symptoms came up like moderate fever, moderate attacks of tetany [a nervous affliction that can include numbness and tingling in the extremities], reintensification of asthma and eczema. This was followed by general improvement.
>
> The asthma vanished and the Lomudal treatment was stopped for good in November 1988, nine months after treatment began. Since then, this patient has not suffered from a single attack of asthma.[6]

AHIT has been used in Germany since 1987 to treat patients suffering from bronchial asthma. Dr. Horst Kief, the developer of AHIT, reported a study on sixty-five patients who were treated over a period of seven months. Dr. Kief found marked improvement in many patients, as indicated by a sharp decrease in, or complete elimination of, the medications they required to control asthma flares. Table 7.1 summarizes the results of his study.

Dr. Kief added: "It may be very encouraging that the consumption of systemic corticoids could be reduced by almost 90% (relative to the exclusive administration of this drug group) and of inhalant cortisone derivatives by more than 85%."[7]

Burns

In a Cuban study of twenty-five patients suffering severe burns at the Calixto García Hospital in Havana, ozone was given in the form of autohemotherapy over the course of ten days. Ozone normalized levels

Table 7.1   Asthma Medication Use

Medication	Patients Using Medication			
	Before AHIT		After AHIT	
	No.	(%)	No.	(%)
Anti-allergic drugs	13	(20)	2	(3.1)
Mediator antagonists	21	(32.3)	8	(12.3)
Secretolytic drugs	19	(29.2)	7	(10.8)
Theophylline derivatives	25	(38.5)	15	(23.1)
Beta-2 agonists	46	(70.8)	12	(18.5)
Systemic cortisone derivatives	35	(53.8)	4	(6.2)
Inhalant cortisone derivatives	28	(43.1)	4	(6.2)

Source: Horst Kief, "Die Behandlung des Asthma bronchiale mit der auto-homologen Immuntherapie (AHIT)," Erfahrungsheilkunde 9 (1990).

of immunoglobulin G and M, complement C4, and antithrombin III—three indicators of greater immune response. The researchers concluded that those results were due to the anti-inflammatory, immunoregulatory, and bacteriocidal qualities of ozone.[8]

Candida

For over ten years, Charles H. Farr has successfully treated hundreds of patients suffering from candidiasis with intravenous hydrogen peroxide at his clinic in Oklahoma City. In his monograph *The Therapeutic Use of Intravenous Hydrogen Peroxide*, Dr. Farr offers a case history of one of his patients:

Ms. P.M., a 34 y/o w/f [34-year-old white female], has been treated repeatedly over the past 5 years for Chronic Systemic Candidiasis. Her history and symptoms are classic. Her current problems had an onset after several episodes of upper respiratory infections, about 5 years ago, which were treated with large doses of various antibiotics. Following this she had repeated episodes of yeast vaginitis and intermittent problems with diarrhea. These episodes were then followed with the development of chronic fatigue, acne, lethargy, migratory arthralgia [joint pain], frequent headaches, menstrual irregularities, mental confusion, difficulty concentrating and a poor tolerance to environmental and exercise stress.

She was treated with various elimination and rotation diets, nystatin, nizoral, monostat, allergic desensitization, and various natural anti-yeast preparations. Each time the therapeutic modality was changed, she would have a temporary subjective improvement for a few days or weeks [and] then relapse to her pretreatment morbid level. She had been unable to work for over two years and had become totally dependent on her mother for financial and physical support. She often did not feel able to dress or feed herself.

She was started on weekly injections of 250ml of 0.15% H_2O_2 and after two treatments reported a significant improvement in alertness, ability to concentrate and had an improved feeling of well being. After the third treatment, she pointed out how her complexion was improving and her acne was considerably better. A menstrual period, the previous week, had been normal and previous signs of vaginitis had disappeared. Her bowel function was becoming more regular and normal and she was talking about wanting to return to work.

Her 4th, 5th and 6th treatments were scored with continued subjective improvements from her previous complaints. After 8 treatments she was free of symptoms for the first time in 5 years. Objectively she appeared much healthier and had more vitality, smiling and happy for the first time since we saw her as a new patient. When tested for candida sensitization subcutaneously, she now tested a 1 dilution compared to her usual 4 to 6 dilutions during her more morbid times. Two months after her last infusion, she was seeking employment, had redeveloped her self-confidence and had shown no signs of relapse. Follow-up evaluations are continuing.[9]

Diabetes

A study was carried out at the National Institute of Angiology and Vascular Surgery in Havana with forty-seven diabetics who suffered from neuroinfected diabetic foot. Amputation is sometimes required if the patient does not improve. The participants in this study, who had suffered from diabetes for nine to nineteen years, were divided into three groups and were treated for a total of ten days.

Group 1 (sixteen subjects) was given ozone therapy, which consisted of a combination of regular wound cleansing with ozonated water followed by treatment with an ozone bag. Autohemotherapy was also administered. Group 2 (sixteen subjects) was treated externally with cane sugar in the form of a syrup. This folk remedy was applied to the wound. A bandage was applied to keep the syrup in contact with the skin for twenty-four hours. Group 3 (fifteen patients) received oral, parenteral (outside the intestines), and intravenous antibiotics as well as traditional medications applied externally to the wound.

Results were classified simply as "good" or "bad." Good meant that surgery was avoided, while bad indicated that some type of surgical intervention was needed to amputate the infected area.

Treatment	Good		Bad	
Group 1 (ozone therapy)	15	(93.8%)	1	(6.2%)
Group 2 (cane sugar)	13	(81.3%)	3	(18.7%)
Group 3 (antibiotics)	10	(66.7%)	5	(33.3%)

The researchers concluded that ozone therapy was the most effective method of treatment for neuroinfected diabetic foot, while cane sugar was a good alternative when ozone therapy was not available. Conventional treatment with antibiotics was considered the least desirable therapy for this particular symptom.[10]

As in many Western countries, diabetes is a major health problem in Russia. A group of Russian physicians investigated the therapeutic use of medical ozone in treating patients with diabetes and reported their findings at the Second International Symposium on Ozone Applications, which took place in Havana in March 1997.

A total of thirty-eight adults were selected who were diagnosed with diabetes in varying degrees of severity; twenty-two suffered from related health complaints, such as dry mouth, low resistance to infection, and cardiovascular problems. Patients were given intravenous injections of ozonated saline solution, as well as rectal insufflations of oxygen and ozone. The course of therapy lasted for several weeks and included seven to ten treatments, depending on the patient.

All subjects showed improvement over the course of therapy. Many stopped complaining of dry mouth, thirst, frequent urination, itch, and tingling and numbness in the hands and feet. Tests showed a 50 percent average reduction of glucose levels in the blood several hours after the first treatment; after the course of therapy, glucose levels among the patients had dropped an average of 30 percent. This led the majority of the patients to reduce their doses of insulin. Positive dynamics involving lipid spectrum, coagulagram and immunogram, a rise of AOA of blood, and lowering of POL products were found as well. The researchers concluded that: "Ozone therapy may be used in a complex treatment of people suffering from diabetes and allows to lower doses of the uses of sugar reduced preparations."[11]

Duodenal Ulcer

At the General Calixto García Hospital in Havana, twenty patients suffering from duodenal ulcer were treated several times daily with ozonated water over the course of one month. Clinical studies revealed that 40 percent of the patients were totally healed by the end of treatment, 10 percent were in the final stages of scar formation, 25 percent had 50 percent scar formation, 5 percent experienced 33 percent scar formation, and 20 percent had to discontinue the study because of intense pain.[12]

Eye Diseases

As in other areas of medical research, Polish physicians have explored the medical value of ozone therapy in treating a wide range of eye problems, including retinal pigment dystrophy, glaucomatous optic atrophy, optic neuritis, eye injuries, degenerative atrophic changes of the choroid, severe myopia, in postinflammatory cases, other degenerative diseases, bacterial corneal ulcerations, and in cases of unknown etiology. A 1992 article reported the preliminary general findings concerning 206 patients with eye problems. Autohemotherapy was performed on 174 patients, and the remaining 32 patients were given intra-arterial oxygen and ozone injections. The researchers observed an improvement in both visual acuity and the visual field. The report added: "Ozone therapy in these conditions seems to be favorable, especially when the pathological process is not extensive."[13]

However, the most exciting research in ozone therapy to treat eye diseases has taken place in Cuba. Over the past few years, Cuban scientists have pioneered research in developing treatment protocols for eye diseases with ozone therapy. Studies evaluated the beneficial effects of ozone for treating glaucoma, corneal ulcers, retinitis pigmentosa, atrophy of the optic nerve, and diabetic retinopathy. Ozone was also studied as an adjunct to corneal transplant operations.

Glaucoma

Glaucoma is a serious disease that affects approximately 2 percent of adults over forty years of age. However, in some countries, up to 11 percent of adults can suffer from glaucoma, making it the third leading cause of blindness in the world. Cuban research evaluating the therapeutic effectiveness of ozone to treat glaucoma was reported at the Twelfth World Congress of the International Ozone Association in 1995. Conducted by scientists at both the Ozone Research Center and the Carlos J. Finlay Hospital in Havana, two hundred outpatients suffering from different stages of simple chronic glaucoma were studied. Ninety percent of patients were over forty years of age.

After being tested for visual acuity, visual field, slit lamp examination, fundoscopy, and visual evoked potentials, patients were divided into three random groups for fifteen daily treatments: those receiving ozone therapy (through rectal insufflation), patients receiving magnetotherapy, and those receiving both ozone therapy and magnetotherapy. After the course of treatment, patients were subjected to the same battery of examinations as before.

Visual acuity results were basically similar among all groups, although those receiving ozone therapy alone scored several percentage points higher: Overall, 71–75 percent of patients showed "highly significant" improvement while 25–29 percent showed "significant" improvement. However, visual field results showed that ozone therapy is more effective: 73 percent of patients receiving ozone therapy alone showed "highly significant improvement" while 27 percent had "significant" improvement; 58 percent of those receiving magnetotherapy alone experienced "highly significant" improvement while 42 percent showed "significant improvement"; 67 percent of patients using combined therapies had "highly significant improvement" while the remaining 33 percent experienced "significant" improvement.

Overall, the researchers found that best results were attained through ozone therapy alone. They also noted that a fifteen-treatment course of ozone therapy worked best with patients suffering from the earlier stages of the disease.[14]

Optic Atrophy

Optic nerve dysfunction, or optical atrophy, is a leading cause of blindness in Cuba. A preliminary study with forty patients (sixty-seven eyes) was carried out at the Institute of Neurology and Neurosurgery in 1992. One treatment of autohemotherapy with ozone was given every weekday for three weeks.

A number of standardized tests were administered before and after the course of treatment, including visual acuity (VA), visual field by Goldman Perimetry measurements (VF), visual evoked potentials (VEP), and Pelli Robson Contact Sensitivity Test (PRCST). The results were as follows:

Test	Percentage patients improved
VA	54.5
VF	82.7
VEP	37
PRCST	85.7

While not all patients achieved a total cure with ozone therapy, the results of this preliminary study so impressed the head physician on the research team (teams are usually composed of chemists, physicians, and technicians) that she decided to treat all of her future patients suffering from optic atrophy with ozone, either alone or as an adjunct to other treatments.[15]

Optic Nerve Dysfunction

A team of researchers at the Institute of Neurology and Neurosurgery in Havana investigated the healing potential of ozone therapy on patients diagnosed with optic nerve dysfunction (OND).

Sixty patients with OND were given a total of fifteen autohemotherapy sessions over a three-week period. Ophthalmological tests to determine visual acuity, visual field by Goldmann Perimetry, visual evoked potentials, and Pelli Robson Contrast Sensitivity Test were done before and after treatment.

The most positive findings were found in PRCST and visual field parameters, indicating improvement in 86 and 83 percent of patients respectively. Visual acuity improved in 55 percent of the patients, while visual evoked potentials increased in 37 percent of patients. No improvement was found in patients diagnosed with Leber optic atrophy.[16]

Retinal Maculopathy

Retinal maculopathy affects the muscles of the eye and often appears in one's later years. The effects of oxygen–ozone therapy on twenty patients affected by age-related degenerative maculopathy was studied by Dr. E. Riva Sanseverino and his colleagues at the University of Bologna. Before-and-after tests to determine visual acuity and eye fluorangiography were used to evaluate the efficacy of the therapy. Ozone was administered via major autohemotherapy at 1500 to 2000 µg/per session over a four-month period. The results were very heartening: Tests indicated that "the majority of patients showed an improvement of their ocular condition, suggesting continuation of this type of investigation on a larger group of people."[17]

Retinitis Pigmentosa

One of the major successes of the Cuban medical system has been in treating retinitis pigmentosa, a chronic progressive disease involving atrophy of the optic nerve and widespread pigmentary changes of the retina. Blindness is often the result. The first major study was carried out in 1985 with a total of two hundred patients (with a range of tubular vision of 5 degrees or less) at the Salvador Allende Hospital in Havana. Believing that ozone might be able to help restore blood circulation to the capillaries of the retina, activate protective enzyme systems, and stimulate metabolism of oxygen, researchers gave the patients either major autohemotherapy or intramuscular treatments of ozone and oxygen daily for fifteen to twenty days, depending on the individual and the severity of symptoms. The patient was said to improve when the range of vision increased to between 10 and 20 percent.

The results were surprising. Of the 175 patients in the study who received autohemotherapy, 112 showed "notable improvement," 45 had "slight improvement," and 18 experienced "no progression of symptoms," meaning that although they did not get better, they also did not get worse. The figures for the 25 patients receiving intramuscular oxygen and ozone injections were 12, 9, and 4, respectively. While a complete cure was not achieved, marked improvement took place in 89 percent of the patients, which persisted for at least two years after treatment. Figure 7.1 offers a view of one patient's visual range before and one year after ozone therapy was administered.[18]

Figure 7.1. Diagram showing range of vision (in white) of patient with retinitis pigmentosa before and after ozone therapy. (From Revista CENIC 20, no. 1–2–3, 1989.)

A later study was carried out at several hospitals in the city of Holguín as part of a larger research project encompassing other ophthalmological diseases. Eighty patients with nonsystemic Stage I and II retinitis pigmentosa were given daily ozone therapy via rectal insufflation for a period of twenty days. Clinical evaluation was made every three months for one year after therapy.

A total of 75 percent realized clinical improvement in their visual acuity up to six months after treatment. However, after one year, only 23 percent of patients maintained this improvement. Regarding visual field, 75 percent of the patients improved after treatment and up to nine months, but after a year, 59 percent maintained their level of improvement. These results led the researchers to recommend that follow-up ozone treatments be scheduled every six months to maintain patient improvement.[19]

These results reflected the opinions of researchers who completed an ongoing ten-year study of twenty patients at the National Reference Center of Retinitis Pigmentosa of the Salvador Allende Hospital in Havana. They wrote: "The best results were achieved when ozone treatment is repeated, at least twice a year, among all these years, with improvement of 70% in the visual field and 42% in the visual acuity."[20]

By the end of 1997, an estimated four thousand patients had been treated with ozone at the hospital for a variety of eye diseases. It is given routinely to the majority of patients with retinitis pigmentosa, retinitis diabetica, keratitis, corneal ulcers, and other eye diseases, either alone or as an adjunct to traditional medical therapies. For retinitis pigmentosa patients, follow-up applications of ozone therapy are recommended twice a year.[21]

Gastroenteritis

Robert Mayer, M.D., a Miami pediatrician, used medical ozone to treat children suffering from gastroenteritis, an inflammation of the stomach and intestinal tract. Nonbacterial diarrhea was a common symptom.

A total of 2757 children, aged one month to eighteen years, were divided into two groups: Group 1 consisted of 1932 children who were treated with oxygen and ozone through rectal insufflation. Of that total, 1265 received one treatment, 583 were given two treatments, and 84 received three treatments. Group 2 was a control group of 825, which was in turn divided into three subgroups: subgroup A received a restricted diet only, subgroup B received rectal air insufflation, and members of subgroup C were given rectal oxygen insufflation.

Of the children receiving ozone therapy, 95 percent of the group receiving one treatment were cured in one day. Of the subjects receiving two treatments, 95 percent were cured in two days. All of the remaining patients receiving ozone were cured in three days. In contrast, all members of the control group recovered more slowly and persisted in their symptoms for up to six days.[22]

Giardiasis

Giardia lamblia is a parasite that can infest the small intestine. For those unfortunate enough to contract this parasitic disease (giardiasis), symptoms include diarrhea, weight loss, nausea, cramps, and vomiting. *Giardia lamblia* is often highly resistant to medical therapy. While giardiasis is usually managed with drugs, there is no known cure.

At the General Calixto García Hospital, fifty adults suffering from giardiasis (who did not respond to traditional medical treatment) were given two cycles of therapy with ozonated water over a twenty-seven-day period. Each patient drank four glasses of ozonated water per day for ten days, which was followed by a seven-day period without treatment. The second cycle consisted of another ten days of drinking four glasses of ozonated water daily.

Researchers reported that twenty-three patients (46 percent) experienced a remission of symptoms during the first cycle of treatment, while twenty-four others (48 percent) became asymptomatic by the end of the second cycle. Unlike many receiving drug therapy, subjects reported no adverse side effects from ozone. The researchers concluded, "Ozone's easy availability and low cost, as well as its great effectiveness in the treatment of *Giardia lamblia,* permits its recommendation to be used on a greater scale and to substitute it for conventional treatments used to treat giardia."[23]

After the success of the previous investigation, a group of researchers from the Ozone Research Center developed a study with physicians from the Department of Parasitology at the Central Havana Pediatric Hospital to see whether ingestion of ozonated sunflower oil could help cure giardiasis in children.

A group of 222 children aged seven months to fourteen years diagnosed with infantile giardiasis were selected for the study. Seventy-six percent (169) of the patients had been previously treated with antigiardastic medications, without success. Children were given drops or capsules of ozonated sunflower oil (it is marketed as Oleozon-A in Cuba) at age-dependent doses at bedtime over a ten-day period. After a break of ten days, another ten-day course of therapy took place.

After the second course of treatment, a duodenal gavage (a procedure using a stomach tube) was performed and feces were examined. The absence of cysts or trophozoites of *Giardia lamblia* in feces and the duodenal gavage would indicate a cure. The results were very encouraging: 79 percent of the patients treated with Oleozon–A were cured. Of the remaining 21 percent, nine out of ten children reported a disappearance of all symptoms, of which abdominal pain and diarrhea were most common. A third cycle of treatment for the noncured patients brought further improvement. No adverse reactions to the therapy were observed.[24]

Gynecological Infections

Over a dozen clinical studies had been carried out in Cuba by 1990 regarding the effects of ozonated sunflower oil on a variety of gynecological infections, including leucorrhea, herpes, and vulvovaginitis.

One such study took place at the Pasteur Polyclinic in Havana with a group of sixty women suffering from vulvovaginitis. A total of 97 percent also had Candida albicans, trichomoniasis, and cardenela vaginalis.

Thirty patients were treated with ozonated sunflower oil, twenty received normal medical therapy, and the remaining ten were given a placebo consisting of oil without ozone. The criteria for cure were determined by examination with a colposcope, a special instrument used to examine the vagina and cervix.

All of the patients who used ozonated oil were completely cured within five to seven days. In the control group, 20 percent were cured within ten to fifteen days. All of the subjects receiving the placebo experienced a worsening of symptoms.[25]

Other studies have been carried out in Russia. One study at the Department of Obstetrics and Gynecology at the Sechenov Medical Academy in Moscow evaluated the effectiveness of ozone on 112 women suffering from a variety of infections, including inflammation of the fallopian tubes, genital herpes, condyloma (wartlike growths on the genitals), and pelvic peritonitis. Depending on the case, patients received 2–5 mg of injectable ozone daily, topical applications of ozonated oil, or irrigation or intra-abdominal injections of ozonated solutions at a concentration of 4–6 mg/ml. The treatments brought substantial relief, leading the doctors to declare that ozone has strong immunomodulative, antiviral, and analgesic properties.[26]

Research into the effectiveness of ozone on acute condyloma was undertaken at the same institute with fifty-three women. They were given eight to ten local applications of different ozonated solutions, such as oil and water. Symptoms in all patients disappeared by the end of treatment. All but two patients remained free of symptoms after eight months. One of the two was retreated and never experienced condyloma symptoms again.[27]

Hearing Loss

When I visited Cuba in 1994, I was introduced to Ernesto Basabe, M.D., an ear, nose, and throat specialist. After meeting him at Cira García Central Clinic in Havana, he took me to the Lina Odena Special School for children with hearing problems. At the time, he was working with thirty-four children suffering from sensoneural hearing loss, scientifically known as *ototoxicity*. Believing that improved circulation in the inner ear may improve hearing, he decided to explore the value of ozone therapy to combat hearing loss in children.

Dr. Basabe and his colleagues divided the students into two random groups. One group received ozone therapy through rectal insufflation over a three-week period, while the other group was given insufflations of oxygen. Careful evaluations of both ears of each child (including audiometry, audio evoked brain–stem potentials (AEBSP), and psycho-pedagogical tests) were made before and after the therapy.

Children who received ozone (thirty-four ears) the "grave level" improved in twenty-three ears (68 percent) and the conversational level improved in nineteen ears (56 percent). In the "acute level," nine ears (26 percent) improved, but not significantly. Among those treated with oxygen (thirty-four ears), no improvement was noted. However, a one-year follow-up found that improvement tended to decrease in roughly half of the patients receiving ozone. For that reason, Dr. Basabe recommended follow-up ozone therapy within a year of the initial course of treatment.

The medical–psychopedagogical integration results showed that eleven (6 percent) of the children receiving ozone improved while six (25 percent) remained the same. Two patients (12 percent) receiving oxygen showed improvement while fifteen (88 percent) remained the same.[28]

Although not a miracle cure, ozone therapy was found to both increase hearing levels and improve overall scholastic efficiency among many of the children receiving ozone therapy. While no adverse side effects were reported, it was among this group that one student, who happened to be suffering from chronic asthma, was completely cured of his symptoms, to the delight of his parents and teachers.

Hepatitis

Among the first physicians to treat hepatitis with medical ozone therapy was Dr. Heinz Konrad of São Paulo, Brazil. During the 1970s he began a study of fifteen adults suffering from acute type A hepatitis and seven adults with chronic type B hepatitis. Major autohemotherapy was administered twice a week.

The most significant improvement took place among those with hepatitis A: 80 percent (twelve patients) recovered after an average of five ozone applications, while three patients required an average of eleven treatments. The latter three were also given steroids after the course of ozone therapy was completed.

Hepatitis B proved more problematic. Treatment was successful in four cases (57.1 percent) and unsuccessful in three cases (42.9 percent). The patients who recovered received an average of 8.1 ozone treatments. Nevertheless, Dr. Konrad felt (in 1982) that medical ozone therapy had "more success and less side-effects than any other method available today."[29]

A more recent study was undertaken by Cuban physicians at the Octavio de la Concepción y de la Pedraja Hospital in Camagüey in cooperation with researchers from two other Cuban health agencies. Eighty patients between the ages of seventeen and forty-five diagnosed with hepatitis A, B, and C were chosen for the study. Conventional treatment (which consisted primarily of bed rest and a special diet) and fifteen sessions of ozone therapy via rectal insufflation was given to forty patients. The other group received conventional therapy only.

The doctors reported that patients receiving ozone saw their symptoms go into remission during the first week and were diagnosed as cured at the end of the three-week trial. The control group began to experience a remission of symptoms after ten days and were diagnosed as cured approximately six months later. Presenting their findings at the Second International Symposium on Ozone Applications, which was held in Havana in March 1997, the researchers concluded: "Comparing these results we can say that ozone therapy is a suitable treatment against hepatitis, improving the patients' health and the healing time of the disease."[30]

There is also clinical evidence that hydrogen peroxide infusions can treat patients suffering from hepatitis C. A paper presented at the International Bio-Oxidative Medicine Association Conference in 1995 by Ronald M. Davis, M.D., described treating thirty-eight-year-old man with hydrogen peroxide who had been experiencing symptoms of hepatitis three months before actually being disgnosed with hepatitis C. The hydrogen peroxide IVs consisted of 0.03 percent solution mixed by giving 2.5 cc of 3 percent hydrogen peroxide in 250 cc D5W (saline solution), with 1.5 cc $NaHCO_3$ (sodium bicarbonate) added. The infusions were administered over a two-hour period.

Dr. Davis reported that the first infusion was given on September 8, 1995, and three days later the patient noted a slight worsening of nausea and fatigue. However, after the second infusion, symptoms began to improve. Symptoms of fatigue, anorexia, and weight loss resolved and the patient (an air-conditioning repairman) returned to work after the fourth treatment. Dr. Davis reported that ". . . laboratory findings went from originally grossly abnormal to entirely normal after a dozen IV hydrogen peroxide treatments over a ten month time-span. This patient was last seen in the office [in] March 1996. He is in good health, feels well and has no complaints. One year after initiating treatment the patient is free of symptoms, feels well, and is at work full time."[31]

Humoral Immune Deficiency

A group of researchers at the Havana Central Pediatric Hospital sought to evaluate the effects of ozone therapy on children with humoral immunity deficiency. A group of fifty-nine children between one and five years of age who had not responded to conventional immune-stimulating therapies were chosen for the study.

Clinical manifestations of patients were as follows:

Frequent recurrence of respiratory infections: 3 patients (6 percent)

Chronic adenoiditis and or tonsillitis: 10 patients (17 percent)

Pneumonia: 22 patients (37 percent)

Asthma: 15 patients (25 percent)

Chronic diffused middle otitis (ear infection): 9 patients (15 percent)

Sepsis: 1 patient (2 percent)

Immunoglobulins are proteins that are capable of acting as antibodies to protect the body from disease. All patients in the study were deficient in one or more immunogloblins: forty-eight (81 percent) patients were deficient in gamma A [IgA], which helps protect mucosal surfaces from invading pathogens; eight (14 percent) were deficient in gamma M [IgM], which is formed in almost all the body's immune responses; and thirty (51 percent) were deficient in gamma G [IgG], the principal immunoglobulin found in human serum.

Immunological improvement was rated as "satisfactory" when immunological studies were normalized or were higher than reference values. They were rated "unsatisfactory" when the immunological parameters remained pathological. Clinical improvement was "satisfactory" when recurrent infectious episodes were relieved or eliminated and "not satisfactory" when infectious episodes continued or increased.

Ozone was administered via rectal insufflation at age-dependent doses in three different cycles. The first cycle included fifteen daily treatments over a three-week period, the second cycle included twelve sessions over six weeks, and the third cycle called for nine ozone insufflations over six weeks, with a break of fifteen days between cycles.

The results were impressive. Researchers found that humoral immunity levels increased while clinical improvements were achieved to a satisfactory level in all patients. In addition, pathological IgA, IgM, and IgG values were normalized within the first cycle of treatment. Finally, the researchers noted that the ozone therapy was well tolerated by all patients and no adverse side effects were present.[32]

Influenza

Many of us have experienced influenza at least once. Symptoms of fever, coughing, chills, body aches, sore throat, headache, and nausea are familiar to many flu sufferers. Some people—especially among the elderly—die from it.

We mentioned earlier that the first known treatment using intravenous hydrogen peroxide for influenza was reported by Dr. T. H. Oliver in the British medical journal *The Lancet* in 1920. Since that time, hydrogen peroxide has been a valuable yet little-known treatment for this common, debilitating, and sometimes fatal disease.

A study to examine the effectiveness of intravenous hydrogen peroxide in treating patients with type A/Shanghai influenza was undertaken by Dr. Charles Farr in January 1989. Symptoms of that strain of flu are very pronounced and typically last for forty-eight to seventy-two hours. Full recovery takes an average of twelve to fifteen days.

Dr. Farr divided a group of forty flu sufferers between the ages of sixteen and seventy-eight into two groups of twenty so that age and gender were similar. The control group received the conventional medical protocol for influenza, which included antibiotics, decongestants, and painkillers. Some patients supplemented those medications with over-the-counter cold and cough preparations of their choice. The treatment group was given 250 ml of 0.0375 percent intravenous hydrogen peroxide over a period of one to three days, according to the patient's needs. Painkillers were also given if desired. Of that group, 35 percent required a second infusion, and two patients (10 percent) needed a third.

The results were impressive. Half of the control group got better after 4.1 days, and 75 percent improved in 7.8 days, with 90 percent reporting improvement after 11 days. Of the group treated with hydrogen peroxide, half got better in 1.9 days, 75 percent in 3.2 days, while 90 percent experienced a complete recovery after only 5.5 days. Overall, the group receiving hydrogen peroxide lost a cumulative 5 days of work, while the controls were absent for a cumulative 41.5 days. Figure 7.2 displays the results in more detail.

Given that millions of North Americans come down with different varieties of influenza every flu season, the time, suffering, and money lost to absenteeism saved through hydrogen peroxide therapy could be significant indeed.[33]

Lyme Disease

Lyme disease has become a major health problem in rural and suburban areas in the United States. Caused by a bacterium passed on to

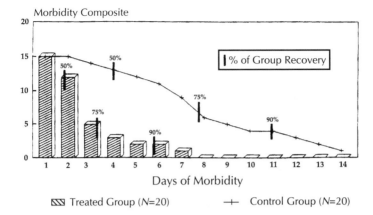

Figure 7.2. Morbidity profiles of Type A/Shanghai influenza. Treated group IV: H_2O_2/analgesic. Control: Antibiotic/decongestant/analgesic). Treated group given 250 ml 0.0375% H_2O_2 first day. Seven required repeat treatments second day. Two required a third. (Reprinted courtesy of Dr. Charles H. Farr.)

humans through the bite of a deer tick, Lyme disease is a multisystemic persistent disease that produces a wide range of symptoms, including chronic fatigue, joint pain, dizziness, sore throat, sleep disturbances, memory loss, headache, and abdominal pain.

In a talk presented at the Eighth International Conference on Bio-Oxidative Medicine in 1997, Kenneth Bock, M.D., a physician from Dutchess County, New York, and author of *The Road to Immunity,* spoke of his experience in successfully treating over a thousand patients suffering from Lyme disease, many referred to him by other physicians.

Although Dr. Bock finds that an aggressive course of antibiotics works best at the onset of Lyme disease, he finds that a combination of alternative modalities including hydrogen peroxide, hyperbaric oxygen therapy, immune-boosting herbs, and nutritional supplements are more useful in treating chronic and "late" Lyme disease. In his talk, Dr. Bock stressed the importance of a careful medical diagnosis in determining the nature and extent of the malady and the need to continue bio-oxidative and other treatments for five weeks or more, even if symptoms disappear. Dr. Bock concluded that "oxidative modalities offer much promise for treatment of these patients with recurrent and/or chronic Lyme disease."[34]

Malaria

Studies at the Middlesex Hospital Medical School in England revealed that blood-stage murine malaria parasites were killed in vitro by hydrogen peroxide at even tiny concentrations. In vivo studies (on mice) showed that hydrogen peroxide was able to kill the lethal varieties of *Plasmodium yoelii* and *P. bergher,* although the latter proved more difficult. The researchers concluded, "We propose that hydrogen peroxide is in fact a possible contributor to the destruction of at least some species of malaria parasite."[35]

Like many other laboratory findings regarding the therapeutic properties of hydrogen peroxide, studies on human beings suffering from malaria have not been done. Given the prevalence of malaria in tropical countries (many strains of which have become resistant to traditional antimalarial drugs), hydrogen peroxide therapy—whether alone or as an adjunct to traditional medications—offers promise to help heal thousands of infected people yearly.

Miscarriage

An unusual Russian study was undertaken by physicians at the Medical Academy in Nizhni Novgorod to determine whether ozone therapy could help pregnant women avoid miscarriage. One hundred ten pregnant women were selected for the study. All had previous miscarriages and were determined to be in danger of another miscarriage by their physicians. Terms of pregnancy ranged from eight to twenty-two weeks.

After a complete physical exam, it was found that many of the women had low levels of several important hormones, including estriol, progesterone, placental lactogen, and cortisol. They also discovered that many had poor immune levels, indicated in part by low phagocytic activity and deficient IgM levels in the blood. Some of the expectant mothers also suffered from hormonal imbalances, infections like clematises, and immune disorders.

Ozone therapy was provided by intravenous applications of 0.9 percent ozonized sodium chloride (NaCl) solutions. A total of five infusions were given over a five-day period.

The results were very encouraging. The researchers found that:

1. Fetoplacental hormones (including oestriol, progesterone, placental

lactogen, prolactin, and cortisol) in the blood became normalized;

2. immune levels improved, as evidenced by normalized levels of phagocytic stimulation and immune complexes in the blood;

3. lipid peroxidation normalized, which appeared to help preserve the membranes of the placenta's cells from free radical damage.

Pregnancy was conserved in 89 percent of the women, who gave birth to healthy babies. The researchers concluded: "We didn't note any complications. . . . This allows us to recommend ozone in appropriate dose[s] for the treatment of the sick with threatened abortion of I–III trimester of pregnancy."[36]

Mouth Diseases

Three percent hydrogen peroxide has long been a popular and inexpensive home remedy for certain diseases of the mouth, taken either full strength or diluted in water. Today, a number of commercial toothpastes and mouthwashes contain hydrogen peroxide.

It was not until 1979 that a university-sponsored study was published in the *Journal of Clinical Periodontology* testifying to hydrogen peroxide's outstanding ability to retard the development of plaque and gingivitis, two of our most common dental problems. Fourteen dental students at the Department of Periodontology at the University of Gothenburg in Sweden took part in this double-blind study. After a thorough dental examination, half of the students were given a mouthwash containing hydrogen peroxide, while the other group was given a placebo mouthwash. The students were told to rinse their mouths three times daily, after meals. Tooth brushing during this two-week trial was not permitted. Measurements of plaque and gingival "index scores" were performed after four, seven, and fourteen days of the trial. Bacteria from the mouth were microscopically examined and analyzed after the first and second weeks.

The results showed that the mouthwash containing hydrogen peroxide effectively prevented the colonization of a number of types of bacteria (including filaments, splrochetes, fusiforms, and motile and curved rods) in developing plaque. It also retarded plaque formation and "significantly retarded" gingivitis development. The researchers concluded, "It is suggested that H_2O_2 released by mouthwashes during rinsing may prevent or retard the colonization and multiplication of anaerobic bacteria."[37]

Over the past few years, a number of toothpaste manufacturers have been marketing toothpaste that is either made with or produce hydrogen peroxide. This led the same Dr. Marshall and his colleagues to review the safety of adding hydrogen peroxide to commercial toothpastes and report their findings in the September 1995 issue of the *Journal of Periodontology.*

The researchers found that daily exposure to the low levels of hydrogen peroxide present in dentifrices is much safer than that to bleaching agents that contain or produce high levels of hydrogen peroxide for an extended period of time. They also reviewed studies in which 3 percent hydrogen peroxide or less was used daily for up to six years, which showed occasional transitory irritant effects in only a small number of subjects with pre-existing ulceration or when high levels of salt solutions were administered at the same time. They also pointed out that if mishandled, bleaching agents that employ or generate high levels of hydrogen peroxide or organic peroxides can produce localized oral toxicity following sustained exposure.

In patients, they found that prolonged use of hydrogen peroxide decreased plaque and gingivitis. However, therapeutic delivery of hydrogen peroxide to prevent gum disease required professional cleaning at the dentist's office. However, they added that "wound healing following gingival [gum] surgery was enhanced due to the antimicrobial effects of topically administered hydrogen peroxide. For most subjects, beneficial effects were seen with H_2O_2 levels above 1%."[38]

In former East Germany, a team of dental researchers investigated the germicidal value of hydrogen peroxide rinses in treating root canal patients suffering from osteitis, or bone inflammation. Thirty-two teeth with the diagnosis of periapical osteitis (established by clinical and radiological examinations) were subjected to irrigation with hydrogen peroxide, followed by bacteriological examinations. The timing of treatment termination depended solely upon clinical evaluation. The examination of smears taken before the last irrigation showed that twenty-six of the thirty-two root canals (81 percent) were germ free; in two cases, an anaerobic infection continued to persist, and in four cases an aerobic infection was observed. Enterococci proved to be the most resistant bacteria to hydrogen peroxide.

The researchers pointed out that "the high percentage of root canals which were germ-free before the last irrigation testifies to the efficiency of hydrogen peroxide application for disinfecting root canals on the one hand, and demonstrates the good agreement between clinical and bacteriological findings on the other hand." They concluded: "The conservative treatment of periapical osteitis by means of root-canal disinfection with a hydrogen peroxide preparation and subsequent root-canal filling with a calcium peroxide paste is recommended."[39]

Neurodermatitis

A significant percentage of the patients seeking care at the Kief Clinic in Germany suffer from neurodermatitis, a chronic and disfiguring autoimmune disease that manifests as eczema, skin rashes, skin eruptions, and intense itching, causing severe physical and emotional distress. There are known genetic and emotional factors to this disease, and it affects people of all ages, from very young children to elderly adults. The symptoms of many of the patients who visit the Kief Clinic do not respond to traditional medical therapies such as corticosteroids.

In a statistical study carried out at the clinic, 115 patients suffering from neurodermatitis were given AHIT over a period of three months. Treatment consisted of injections and oral medication for the adults, while children were given oral AHIT only.

The results, published in the medical journal *Erfahrungsheilkunde* in 1989, were classified as follows: "Full remission" was described as being totally free of symptoms until the study was published two and a half years after treatment; "significantly improved" included greatly improved skin symptoms with a corresponding decrease or disappearance of itching; "improvement" meant that skin conditions got better and/or itching was relieved. Under those classifications, forty-three patients (37 percent) had full remission, fifty (44 percent) showed significant improvement, and thirteen (11 percent) improved. Seven patients (6 percent) did not respond to therapy, while two (2 percent) experienced a worsening of symptoms over the long term.[40]

The results of a more recent study of 333 individuals with neurodermatitis (blindly selected from a total of 2254) were reported by Dr. Kief in the March 1993 issue of *Erfarungsheilkunde*. Patients with multiple symptoms, such as those of neurodermatitis and asthma, were included.

Kief's findings were consistent with the earlier results regarding long-term remission. However, they demonstrated a temporary full remission of 65 to 67 percent, which represented an increase over the 1989 study.[41] "Before" and "after" photos of two of Dr. Kief's patients are reproduced in figure 7.3.

Orthopedic Problems

A study of the value of ozone therapy in treating orthopedic problems was undertaken by C. H. Siemsen, M.D., a specialist in orthopedics and sports medicine and a lecturer in Biomedical Technology at the Polytechnic College in Hamburg. Fifty-nine male and female patients were chosen for the study. Patients were suffering from acute and chronic joint diseases, including active inflammatory gonarthrosis, stiffness of the shoulder and shoulder area, and chronic diseases of the shoulder joint with calcification and painful restrictions of movement. Patients also suffered from lateral and medial epicondylitis (tennis elbow), chronic adductor insertion endopathia (known as "footballer's hip" in Europe), and malformations of the hip, including acute and chronic bursitis trochanteria. Ozone treatment was carried out after all other forms of medical therapy were deemed unsuccessful.

Over a period of several weeks, fifty patients were given an average total of ten interarticular injections of ozone and oxygen in the affected areas preceded by a local anaesthetic. Nine patients suffering from therapy-resistant systemic conditions were given a course of autohemotherapy as well. Patients were examined the day after each treatment.

The patients were assessed with scores by adding the numbers 1 to 6 to form quotients: A value of 1.9 (i.e., good) was a measure for the knee joint (activated gonoarthrosis), and a value of 2.5 (i.e., good to satisfactory) was assigned to shoulder joint problems. After the course of treatment, all patients improved to a "good" quotient level. It was noted that none of the patients required corticosteroids. Dr Siemsen concluded that "the application of ozone in orthopedics and in the treatment of acute, chronic or therapy-resistant painful diseases of the joints with involvement or the articular and periarticular regions is a good alternative treatment method for obtaining rapid pain relief, subsidence of inflammation and an increase in motility."[42]

Figure 7.3. Two of Dr. Kief's patients with neurodermatitis, before and after receiving AHIT. (Photos courtesy of Dr. Horst Kief.)

Osteoarthritis

At the Center of Medical-Surgical Studies in Havana, sixty patients with osteoarthritis (mostly affecting the knees) were given one interarticular injection of ozone per week for a total of ten weeks. Of the sixty patients, only four experienced a return of painful symptoms after two months, while the majority (93.3 percent) were symptom free. The researchers concluded that this easily applied and low-cost therapy produced "disappearance of pain after the first several ozone applications, as well as diminished clinical inflammation of the joints and restoration of normal joint movement."[43]

Osteoporosis

Osteoporosis is a degenerative disease involving a lack of calcium and resultant softening of the bones. It primarily affects older women. The effects of ozone therapy in the treatment of patients with osteoporosis were first reported in the journal *Europa Medicophysica* in 1988 by Dr. E. Riva Sanseverino, who conducted the knee-joint study described earlier. A total of 225 women suffering from this disease were studied at the Institute of Human Physiology in Bologna, Italy, over a six-year period.

Dr. Riva Sanseverino and his colleagues divided the patients into three groups: Class A patients (121) received only traditional medical therapy such as hormones, and Class B patients (53) were treated with both drugs and ozone in the form of major autohemotherapy. The forty-three patients making up Class C were treated like those of Class B, except they were given therapeutic exercises to perform on a regular basis. There were originally eight patients in Class D who were treated only with ozone. However, they were soon moved into the B group because the ozone only relieved their pain. (Although pain relief was important, a major focus of the study was on increased bone density.) Members of Class B and Class C were treated with ozone twice a week for six weeks three times a year.

The results revealed that all groups of patients showed improvement in bone density indices, reduction of joint pain, appetite, and ability to sleep. However, it was found that Class B patients experienced a higher degree of bone density than those in Class A, who received traditional medical therapy. They also reported a greater overall sense of well-being in a shorter amount of time than Class A patients and required fewer treatments over the course of the study. Patients who joined Group C did even better. Not only did their bone density indices reach higher levels, but they required less medical treatment over the long term than members of Classes A and B. Dr. Riva Sanseverino concluded:

1. The pharmacological therapy of osteoporosis, if applied alone, helps but is not sufficient to keep the bone tissue at a physiological level of mineralization.

2. The association of oxygen–ozone therapy to the pharmacological one represents a strong potentiation of the above benefit.

3. The latter benefit is further potentiated by the addition of therapeutic exercises, a triad that represents a very powerful tool in particular conditions.[44]

Dr. Kief also has treated patients suffering from osteoporosis. During my visit to his clinic, he spoke of a seventy-two-year-old patient suffering from both immune vascularis (inflammation of the blood vessels) and advanced osteoporosis. The patient was given autohemotherapy to begin with, followed by long-term AHIT, which Dr. Kief believes is more effective.[45] After one year, X rays showed the normal calcification of bones, as seen in figure 7.4.

Figure 7.4. X-ray photographs of a seventy-two-year-old patient with osteoporosis, before and after major autohemotherapy. (Photos courtesy of Dr. Horst Kief.)

Parkinson's Disease

A pioneer study to determine the effectiveness of ozone therapy in the treatment of Parkinson's disease was recently undertaken by researchers at the 10 de Octubre Clinical-Surgical and the Ozone Research Center in Havana. Eighty elderly patients between sixty and seventy-nine years of age diagnosed with Parkinson's syndrome were given fifteen sessions of rectal ozone plus physical therapy over a three-week period. Complete neurological and psychometric exams were given before and after therapy.

According to the researchers' report at the Second International Symposium on Ozone Applications in 1997: "The results demonstrated that all symptoms and signs improved after the treatment, fundamentally the rigidity (95.7%), the gait (95.3%) and the bradiphrasia (88.8%). The Daily Life Activities improved in 95% of the treated patients. [No] side-effect or intolerance were observed during the treatment. In general, an improvement in the quality of life of these patients, increasing their autonomy for a much longer period was achieved."[46]

Peritonitis

Peritonitis is a life-threatening infection affecting the inside wall of the abdomen. At the Scientific Research Institute of Emergency Aid in Moscow, doctors used a mixture of oxygen and ozone on a variety of patients suffering from diffused peritonitis. In a report presented at the First All-Russian Scientific and Practical Conference on Ozone in Biology and Medicine in 1992, they commented: "Ozone therapy . . . caused [an] increase of phagocyte [the cell that kills bacteria and viruses] activity and digestive ability of the leukocytes ["scavenger" white blood cells that fight infection]; hemogram [blood count] indexes improved, the process of healing was accelerated, [and] the period of treatment was reduced."[47]

Physical Activity Enhancement

Because ozone has been found to improve blood flow and enhance oxygen release from cells, Dr. E. Riva Sanseverino and Dr. P. Castellacci from the Institute of Physiology at the University of Bologna sought to evaluate the impact of ozone therapy on physical activity. They took a group of eight healthy adults between forty-two and sixty years of age and tested their endurance on an elevated treadmill for thirty to forty-five minutes, which included both walking and running. Heartbeat and oxygen consumption were measured. The eight individuals were then given ozone through major autohemotherapy once or sometimes twice a week over a four-month period. To establish a control, some were given infusions with added oxygen only. After each treatment, they would be tested on the treadmill and results would be evaluated. Overall, the researchers found that physical performance carried out twelve to twenty-four hours after one to nine sessions of autohemotherapy improved by 8 to 12 percent. Of special note was that the heart rate progressively decreased as the number of autohemotherapy sessions increased.[48]

Plastic Surgery

A team of physicians from the Silesian Medical Academy in Katowice, Poland, explored the benefits of ozone to reduce post operative complications of rhinoplasty (plastic surgery of the nose). A total of forty-five patients were divided into two groups: Twenty-five were given intravenous ozone daily for three days prior to their operation and for three days after the rhinoplasty was performed. The other group of twenty patients did not receive ozone. The researchers reported that ozone therapy was very helpful, "resulting in a significant reduction in post-operative complications duration as compared with the control group. . . ."[49]

Rheumatoid Arthritis

Rheumatoid arthritis is a chronic, systemic disease that causes one's joints to swell and become painful. It is usually treated with anti-inflammatory drugs.

Research at Cuba's Institute of Rheumatology in 1988 compared the effectiveness of ozone and anti-inflammatory drugs on seventeen patients. In that study, doctors administered a very low dose (0.7 mg) of ozone per day intramuscularly to ten patients for eight weeks, while the control group of seven patients was given traditional anti-inflammatory drugs. In all criteria (such as morning stiffness, painful movements, onset of fatigue, strength of handclasp, and joint swelling), the patients who received ozone scored approximately 25 percent better than those receiving drug therapy. In addition, those patients suffered no adverse side effects, while all the nonozonated patients either received additional steroids or suffered symptoms of gastritis.[50]

Approximately 10 percent of patients seeking care at the Kief Clinic suffer from rheumatoid arthritis. In a statistical study of eighty-four such patients receiving AHIT, Dr. Kief reported the following results: 16 percent experienced a full remission of symptoms, 36 percent showed significant improvement (including a decrease in swelling, improved mobility, and less pain), 32 percent experienced some improvement, and 12 percent had no improvement at all.[51]

Senile Dementia

A double-blind study was conducted in the early 1990s at the Department of Geriatrics of the Salvador Allende Hospital in Havana on sixty elderly patients suffering from senile dementia. The first group of thirty received ozone–oxygen therapy via rectal insufflation for twenty-one days, while the second group (the controls) received insufflations of oxygen alone. Before and after the study, all patients were carefully evaluated by clinical examination (including CT scans and electro-encephalograms), psychometrical tests (which measure intelligence, aptitude, behavior, and emotional reactions), and other standardized diagnostic tests for senile dementia.

Among members of the first group, 85 percent of the patients showed overall improvement in their symptoms of vascular and degenerative dementia: Specifically, 73 percent experienced marked improvement in medical status, 83 percent showed improvement in mental condition, 83 percent were better able to self-administer medications, and 80 percent had a greater ability to interact socially and manage daily activities. In contrast, there was no improvement among any of the members of the control group in any of the categories. No adverse side effects were noted among the patients receiving ozone therapy.[52]

Another Cuban study evaluating the long-term benefits of ozone therapy on patients suffering from senile dementia was carried out at the Camilo Cienfuegos Provincial Hospital in Sanci Spiritus. Thirty patients were chosen for the study: All were diagnosed with Alzheimer's dementia, multi-infarction dementia, and vascular epilepsy. Ozone was administered via rectal insufflation over a two-year period. Their findings substantiated the results of the other Cuban studies: Although complete cures were not achieved, clinical improvement was noted in twenty-one patients (70 percent), seven patients (23 percent) remained the same, and two patients (7 percent) got worse.[53]

By 1998, over eight hundred elderly patients had been treated with ozone at the Salvador Allende Hospital. While Cuban physicians do not believe that ozone therapy is a cure for senile dementia, the marked improvement in the overall quality of life of the patients (and their families) has made ozone treatment a standard part of the therapeutic protocol at the Department of Geriatrics. Doctors note greater physical energy among the patients and an improved ability to manage their daily lives. There is also a marked relief of symptoms of depression among patients suffering from Alzheimer's disease.

After an initial two-week cycle of treatment, patients often return to the hospital once a year for an additional week of ozone therapy. No other medications are given.[54]

Sepsis

Sepsis is a highly dangerous and often fatal form of blood poisoning that can occur after accidents or operations. At the Carlos J. Findlay Hospital in Havana, the effectiveness of ozone therapy was studied in the intensive care unit on patients suffering from severe sepsis. It was found that ozone not only increased general oxygen transport to the tissues, the circulatory system, and the respiratory system, it also proved to be an effective germicide. The results of that study led the hospital administration to authorize ozone therapy for accident victims in the intensive care unit of the hospital whenever the risk of sepsis existed.[55]

Sickle Cell Anemia

Sickle cell anemia is a hereditary chronic form of anemia affecting only black people. It is difficult to cure, and its symptoms include episodes of intense pain and fatigue. Believing that ozone could help those suffering from this disease, James A. Caplan of CAPMED/USA, a research organization, originally proposed that a study be done at the Philadelphia Children's Hospital, but he was rebuffed by hospital authorities. Knowing that Cuba has a large African-American population, Caplan offered his proposal to scientists at Cuba's National Center for Scientific Research. The Cubans were glad to collaborate, and the study was undertaken in 1989 at the Salvador Allende Hospital with fifty-five adults.

A control group of twenty-five patients received fifteen conventional medical treatments for sickle cell anemia, while the other group underwent fifteen sessions of oxygen–ozone therapy via rectal insufflation. Some members of the second group also received topical applications of ozone to treat skin ulcers, while patients in the control group were given conventional skin medications.

The results showed that the average time for resolution of the sickle cell crisis among those treated with ozone was half that of the control group. In addition, the frequency and severity of painful crises among the patients receiving ozone diminished during the six-month follow-up in comparison to members of the control group. Skin ulcers, which are common among sickle cell patients, completely disappeared among the patients receiving ozone. The results of this simple, low-cost therapy were so impressive that Cuba's Ministry of Public Health (MINSAP) later approved ozone therapy as a standard treatment for sickle cell anemia throughout the country.[56]

Silicone-Induced Immune Dysfunction Syndrome

Intravenous hydrogen peroxide has recently become an important element in the holistic treatment of silicone-induced immune dysfunction syndrome, a condition that is affecting a growing number of the estimated two million women who have received silicone breast implants since 1962. Although symptoms may not appear for years, this syndrome is believed to cause a wide variety of health problems, including hypersensitivity to food, chemicals, molds, and dust; fatigue; lung problems; anxiety and depression; elevated cholesterol; skin rashes; memory loss; and gastrointestinal problems. While silicone is not believed to be the only cause of those problems, some physicians consider it to be an important aspect of the total environmental load (including pollution, medications, and stress) that depresses the body's overall immune response.

At the Fifth International Conference on Bio-Oxidative Medicine in

1994, environmental medical specialist Stephen B. Edelson, M.D., reported his clinical findings of patients suffering from this syndrome. He administered intravenous hydrogen peroxide one to two times weekly "with great success" as an adjunct to holistic medical therapy, including traditional medication, diet, nutrition, exercise, and other modalities. He called hydrogen peroxide "very, very efficacious," particularly in treating pain and relieving symptoms of chronic fatigue.

Dr. Edelson believes that bio-oxidative therapies like intravenous hydrogen peroxide are useful in treating patients with silicone-induced immune dysfunction syndrome in the following ways:

1. They improve oxidative phosphorylation (phosphorylase is an enzyme in mitochondria, the source of energy in cells involved in protein synthesis and lipid metabolism).

2. They destroy old T-cells, which are then replaced by new, healthier ones. This improves overall immune function.

3. They increase oxygen tissue tensions, making the cells more resistant to oxidation.

4. They aid in hormonal regulation.

5. They aid in the regulation of neurotransmitters.

6. They stimulate enzyme systems.

7. They dilate the small arteries, thus improving blood circulation.

8. They may chemically disrupt the bonds in silicone polymer, making it more difficult for silicone to affect the body.[57]

Although more studies need to be made of the effects of bio-oxidative therapies on this growing health problem, Dr. Edelson's findings reveal the potential value of such therapies as part of a holistic approach to treating disease.

Skin Diseases

A preliminary study of sixty-five patients suffering from one or more of thirteen different skin diseases (including herpes zoster, herpes simplex, eczema, herpes progenitalis, and pyoderma) at Russia's Dermatovenereological Dispensary in Nizhni Novgorod (Gorky) was reported by Dr. S. L. Krivatkin at the Eleventh Ozone World Congress in San Francisco in 1993.

Minor autohemotherapy with ozone was given at different doses and frequencies according to the patient's symptoms. In addition to ozone, traditional medications were given to nineteen patients suffering from acne, eczema, and alopecia, an abnormal baldness affecting different parts of the scalp.

The best results were reported among patients suffering from herpes zoster. There was a total disappearance of symptoms for at least six months in 80 percent of the subjects, with a three-month remission rate among the remaining 20 percent suffering from herpes zoster. A total of twenty-five of the twenty-six patients with pyoderma (any pus-producing skin disease) experienced either complete remission or considerable improvement, with nineteen patients still in remission after six months. All sixteen patients with eczema either were completely cured or showed marked improvement, with a 50 percent remission rate after six months. At the end of his presentation, Dr. Krivatkin commented: "This preliminary research provides every reason to conclude that ozone therapy in practical dermatovenereology produces positive results due to its sufficient therapeutic efficacy, ease of use and safety."[58]

This study was later expanded to a total of 350 patients. It included 60 patients with symptoms of acne and rosacea, alopecia (17 patients), drug-related skin eruptions (3), eczema (52), herpes (70), lichen planus (14), neurodermatitis (22), prurigo (2), psoriasis (27), psoriatic arthritis (8), pyoderma (47), scleroderma (4), tinea pedis (15), and venous leg ulcers (10). Different forms of ozone therapy (such as autohemotherpy, ozone bagging, and intramuscular injection) were applied, depending on the symptoms being treated; in some cases ozone therapy was complemented with traditional allopathic medications.

In his presentation at the Twelfth Ozone World Congress in Lille, France, two years later, Dr. Krivatkin and his colleagues reported that ozone therapy continued to be shown effective in treating skin diseases. Diseases that best responded to ozone therapies (i.e., which most often brought about "complete recovery") included herpes, pyoderma, drug eruptions, and tinea pedis. "Considerable improvement" took place most often in patients with venous leg ulcers, lichen planus, alopecia, neurodermatitis, psoriasis, and eczema. "Improvement" was found mostly in patients suffering from acne, venous leg ulcers, and neurodermatitis, while the patients least responsive to ozone therapy suffered from lichen planus and alopecia. Therapeutic results may be roughly equal in more than one category. For example, six patients suffering from venous leg ulcers enjoyed "considerable improvement" while six showed "improvement." Dr. Krivatkin concluded: "Thus, ozone therapy is effective, almost universal, safe, inexpensive, easy to use and useful in out-patient dermatological practice."[59]

Athlete's Foot

Because of the warm and humid tropical climate, athlete's foot (epidermophytosis) is common in Cuba. It is often resistant to medication and tends to return.

A study of one hundred patients was undertaken at the Pasteur Polyclinic in Havana, with half of the subjects applying ozonized sunflower oil three times a day to the infected area, while the other fifty used traditional antifungal medications. Symptoms cleared up completely within ten to fifteen days for 96 percent of the patients using ozonated oil, while only 20 percent of the control group were cured after fifteen days.[60]

Herpes Simplex

In addition to his pioneer research on the effects of medical ozone on hepatitis, Dr. Heinz Konrad of Brazil is believed to be the first physician to treat herpes with ozone, having shared his experience with other physicians for the first time in 1981. His second study with herpes involved twenty-eight patients suffering from different varieties of herpes simplex: twenty had genital herpes, four had cutaneous (skin) herpes, two had herpes labialis (herpes of the lips), and two suffered from herpes of the eye. Most had been treated unsuccessfully by other physicians.

Dr. Konrad gave all patients 9 mg of ozone in the form of autohemotherapy twice a week for three weeks. Most were given six treatments, although a few received eight or nine treatments. Their progress was monitored for two and a half years after treatment.

The results of the second study, reported in 1982, were impressive, especially among the patients suffering from genital and cutaneous herpes. "Absolute success" was recorded in 85 percent of the patients with genital herpes, while 15 percent reported partial improvement. All of the patients with cutaneous herpes recovered completely. Half of those with oral herpes and half with ophthalmic (eye) herpes recovered completely, while the other half experienced what Dr. Konrad called "questionable success."[61]

Dr. R. Mattassi and his associates at the Division of Vascular Surgery at the Santa Corona Hospital in Milan, Italy, also studied the effects of ozone and oxygen on different varieties of herpes. In one study, they treated twenty-seven patients with herpes simplex labialis with intravenous injections of oxygen and ozone. All patients healed completely after a minimum of one and a maximum of five injections, with a recurrence in only three patients over the next five years. As is usual with ozone therapy, no adverse side effects were reported among any of the participants in the study.[62]

Herpes Zoster

Dr. Mattassi and his colleagues also treated thirty patients with herpes zoster (shingles) at the Santa Corona Hospital in Milan. Herpes zoster is a very painful disease that often takes many weeks to treat. Many patients have trouble sleeping, and some are known to have attempted suicide to escape their intense discomfort.

In the Mattassi study, patients were treated daily with intravenous injections of oxygen and ozone. All of the subjects experienced a complete remission of symptoms of skin lesions after a minimum of five and a maximum of twelve injections. In most cases, local redness disappeared after two to three days of treatment. However, five elderly patients with long-term herpes complained of pain up to two months after therapy, even though their observable symptoms had disappeared.[63]

In a year-long study sponsored by the Center of Medical and Surgical Research (CIMEQ) in Havana, fifteen adults suffering from herpes zoster were treated daily with a combination of ozonated sunflower oil and intramuscular injections over a course of fifteen days. All patients noted marked improvement after only three applications, and by the end of treatment, all patients were judged symptom free. Follow-up inquiries a year later revealed no relapse of symptoms. The researchers concluded: "We can say that this study demonstrates the superiority of treating herpes zoster with ozone over traditional therapies. Its low cost, easy availability and simple application make it preferable to other methods."[64]

In his presentation at the 1983 Ozone World Congress in Washington, D.C., Dr. Heinz Konrad made the following observations on the treatment of herpes zoster with ozone therapy:

> Those few patients I could treat from the very beginning of their herpes zoster experienced a relatively fast recovery. It never took longer than 6

to 8 weeks to get them well and stop the ozone therapy. However, those patients whom I could only treat after they had already had their herpes zoster for weeks or months, or even years, needed a much longer time to feel any better. . . . It seems, thus, of utmost importance, to treat a herpes zoster patient with ozone from the very beginning of his disease in order to have a chance of *complete* recovery.[65]

In 1995, Dr. Konrad presented a paper at the Twelfth Ozone World Congress in France detailing his seventeen years' experience in treating herpes patients with ozone. Of special interest were his findings about the ability of ozone therapy to reduce the "post-zoster neuralgia" (PNZ) pain of individuals suffering from herpes zoster.

Percentage of patients whose pain remained absolutely unchanged: 8

Percentage of patients whose pain was "somewhat" (25 percent) reduced: 4

Percentage of patients whose pain was "significantly" (50 percent) reduced: 28

Percentage of patients whose pain was "mostly" (75 percent) eliminated: 14

Percentage of patients whose pain was totally (100 percent) eliminated: 46

He recalled that the best results were achieved when ozone therapy was combined with the Huneke brothers' "Neuraltherapie" methods introduced early in this century, and stressed that the speedier healing was seen in people who began ozone therapy in the earlier stages of the disease.[66]

Hypodermatitis

A randomized open study of 117 adults suffering from indurative hypodermatitis (a subcutaneous hardening of tissue) or localized lipodystrophy (atrophy of subcutaneous fat) was coordinated by researchers affiliated with the Institute of Pharmacology II at the University of Pavia in Italy.

Participants were divided into two random groups. After careful examination and evaluation, one group of patients was given subcutaneous injections of ozone and oxygen according to established protocols once a week over a five-week period. Members of the control group were given treatments of Essaven gel, a conventional medication, three or more times a day for five weeks. At the end of the trial, both the physician and patient evaluated the efficacy of treatment in terms of "very good," "good," "fair," "poor," and "nil."

Overall, ozone treatments showed a much higher success rate than the gel treatments as seen in the following chart:

	Ozone (%)	Gel (%)
Physician evaluation of treatments		
Very Good	35.1	0.0
Good	59.5	7.5
Fair	5.4	10.0
Poor	0.0	52.5
Nil	0.0	30.0
Patient evaluation of treatments		
Very Good	33.8	0.0
Good	57.1	7.5
Fair	9.1	0.0
Poor	0.0	52.5
Nil	0.0	30.0

The researchers concluded that ". . . oxygen–ozone therapy applied within the limits and with the methods indicated in protocol, leads to a more rapid and more extensive remission of the major objective signs of the pathology (circumference of the affected part and skin temperature) as compared with conventional gel therapy."[67]

Nail Fungus

Onicomycosis is a fungal infection that affects the nails of the hands and feet. It is often highly resistant to traditional medical therapy. A group of researchers from the Ozone Research Center and the Carlos J. Finlay Hospital in Havana studied two hundred adult outpatients suffering from onicomycosis. They were divided into two equal randomized groups: One group received one drop of ozonated sunflower oil (Oleozon) on each sick nail twice a day, while the other group was treated twice a day with tolnaflate solution. The course of treatment lasted three months. Other medications were added for the control patients suffering from yeast infections and filamentous mycosis.

A patient was considered "cured" when the affected nail completely regained normal color, growth, and thickness and no fungi were detected; a patient "improved" when a decrease of symptoms was present and with a positive findings of fungi; "same" symptoms indicated no changes in the nails and a positive finding of fungi; and "worse" when nail lesions increased and fungi was found. The results can be seen in the following table:

Group	Number of patients			
	Worse	Same	Improved	Cured
Experimental	0	0	31	69
Control	0	68	25	7

Researchers concluded that this study demonstrated the fungicidal power of ozonated oil and recommended it as superior to conventional medical treatments. I would like to add that this author's eighty-year-old aunt had suffered from onicomycosis on one nail that was resistant to conventional therapy for over ten years. After applying Oleozon for a week, symptoms completely disappeared.[68]

Warts

Warts are a common skin problem caused by a virus. Physicians often treat warts by cutting, burning, or medicating them. Hydrogen peroxide is a little-known remedy for removing warts painlessly and permanently. The following treatment for warts with 30 percent hydrogen peroxide was described by the German physician Dr. M. Manok in the journal *Hautarzt:*

> One needs a sharp spoon, not to remove the wart, [but] rather to open the surface. One doesn't need to get to the root which would cause it to bleed. . . . With an eyedropper, drop 1 drop of 30% H_2O_2 onto the opened surface and let it dry. After 2 or 3 days scrape off the dried layer and add another drop of H_2O_2. How many times depends on size of the wart. For middle-sized warts it will usually take 4 to 5 applications. Larger ones will take longer. With *Verrucae planea juvenilis,* the most it will take is 2 applications to have it disappear without a trace. Of special importance is, that the plantar wart, which is otherwise hard to remove, can be treated successfully that way. The pain stops mostly after the first or second application. So the patient shouldn't have trouble walking.[69]

Snakebite

In 1983, Robert A. Mayer, M.D., reported on the antitoxic effects of ozone and oxygen at the Sixth Ozone World Congress in Washington, D.C. Having acquired cobra venom from the Miami Serpentarium, Dr. Mayer injected the venom into two groups of mice (no humans came forward to volunteer for this experiment!). One group was given the venom alone, while the other group received an injection of cobra venom mixed with ozone gas. The control group died immediately, while the mice injected with venom and ozone showed no evidence of poisoning. In another test, rattlesnake venom was used, with similar results.

Dr. Mayer also reported the case of a dog (fortunately not a laboratory animal) that was bitten by a rattlesnake in the leg. In addition to two intravenous injections of ozone and oxygen, similar injections were applied around the bite itself. Within thirty-six hours, the dog recovered completely, with no infections of the leg or lymph nodes appearing for the six months the dog was monitored.[70]

Trauma

An unusual study on the effects of ozone therapy on patients suffering from a variety of severe physical traumas was undertaken by researchers from the Center of Ozonotherapy in the intensive care unit at a hospital in Nizhni Novgorod in Russia. The researchers worked with sixteen pediatric patients (between twenty months and fourteen years of age) who were admitted to the emergency room for severe injuries caused by explosions, fires, carbon monoxide poisoning, bullet wounds, and car accidents. All patients suffered obvious damage to the skin, soft tissues, and/or bones.

Over a forty-eight-hour period, one or more types of ozone therapies were utilized on a case-by-case basis. They included tiny amounts of ozone (2–5 µg/liter) added to oxygen for therapeutic inhalation, ozonated sodium chloride given intravenously, major autohemotherapy administration, and ozonated water topically applied to wounds and then drained out. In cases of scalp wounds, open fractures, anaerobic infections, burns, and initial gangrene, ozone was administered through a plastic bag wrapped around the wound. At times, ozonated water or ozone gas was injected directly into bones. Burn victims were sometimes placed in a bathtub containing ozonated water for thirty to forty minutes to speed the healing of damaged tissues.

The researchers found that ozone accelerated the healing of wounds, reduced pain, and prevented necrosis of the tissues. They concluded that ozone therapy can be of significant value in trauma cases, especially in treatment of patients with sepsis and anaerobic infections.[71]

Ozone is generally not recommended for inhalation. However, the Russian researchers found that extremely small amounts of ozone mixed with pure oxygen can be both harmless and beneficial in some cases. It is now considered an accepted adjunct to other therapies in Russia.

Tuberculosis

Studies in Russia have shown that ozone can be an important method of treatment for tuberculosis. One study, carried out by Dr. A. A. Priimak and his colleagues, investigated the impact of a gaseous ozone–oxygen mixture (OOM) on Mycobacterium tuberculosis (MBT) and opportunistic microorganisms. One group of patients was given ozone therapy, while the other group received traditional medical therapy. They found that after fifteen and thirty minutes of exposure, the mixture of ozone and oxygen caused a "significant decrease" in the number of colonies of microorganisms as compared with the controls. They observed that the ozone and oxygen mixture produced the highest effect of MBT suspension, which the researchers felt was probably related to a greater surface of ozone contact with a cell than with a dense medium and higher concentration of ozone and its highly active radicals that arise from the treatment process. Specifically, after treatment with ozone, between 80 and 90 percent of the microbial cells lost their reproductive ability. They also found that the strains grown after ozone and oxygen action retain drug sensitivity of the original strain. The researchers concluded that "the results suggest that the use of a gaseous OOM mixture is promising in the treatment of tuberculosis to cleanse the destruction cavities and pleural empyemas, including those of nonspecific etiology."[72]

Varicose Ulcers

Varicose ulcers are open sores in the extremities found primarily among individuals suffering from diabetes mellitus or varicose veins. The ulcers often get infected and are difficult to treat.

In 1988, scientists at the Pasteur Polyclinic in Havana wondered if the germicidal properties of ozonated oil could stimulate tissue regeneration among patients suffering from varicose ulcers. They chose 120 subjects with varicose ulcers: Half of the patients were treated with ozonated sunflower oil, and the other half (the control group) were given conventional topical medications.

All of the patients using the ozonated oil were completely cured within 15 to 30 days, while the majority of the control group needed an average of 53 days. A few members of the control group had not recovered by the end of the study, which lasted 155 days. In addition to its efficiency, the researchers noted that the patients receiving ozone therapy did not require hospitalization, since the oil could be easily applied at home.[73]

Wound Healing

An early study at the Baylor University Medical Center, reported in the *American Journal of Surgery*, analyzed the ability of intra-arterial hydrogen peroxide to heal wounds, especially those caused by radiation treatment for carcinomas. In the five cases discussed in the article, the researchers found that not only did the wounds heal at a much faster rate and with less scar formation than is normally expected, but the tumors in patients receiving hydrogen peroxide responded more rapidly to irradiation. The researchers attributed the accelerated healing to superoxygenating the irradated area with hydrogen peroxide. They also pointed out that the patients used in the study were unresponsive to conventional modes of therapy for their wounds.

The article also reported how hydrogen peroxide helped speed the healing of other wounds, including a persistent skin ulcer (caused by previous irradiation); athlete's foot; stasis ulcers of the foot, leg, and jaw; varicose ulcers; diabetic ulcers; and a draining osteomyelitis (bone inflammation) of the tibia, all with significant success.[74]

PART III

A HOLISTIC PROTOCOL

Bio-oxidative therapies are an integral part of a holistic approach to health. They assist the body in oxidating viruses and bacteria in addition to weak and sick tissue cells, so that stronger and healthier cells can take their place.

While the use of ozone and hydrogen peroxide by themselves has achieved important results (Cuban physicians, for example, often use ozone alone when treating patients), a growing number of bio-oxidative practitioners are seeing the value of taking a holistic approach to health, one that teaches that to heal the patient, one must address the individual as a whole, including the physical body, the mind, and the spirit. According to Janet F. Quinn, Ph.D., R.N., in her essay "The Healing Arts in Modern Health Care":

> The Holistic Health perspective acknowledges the fundamental whole-
> ness, unity and integrity of the individual in interaction with the environ-
> ment. Body–mind–spirit are viewed as inseparable and interdependent
> dimensions of being. All behaviors, including health and illness, are
> manifestations of the life process of the whole person.[1]

Believing that all aspects of the person are interrelated and that each has an impact on all other aspects of one's being, holistic practitioners address issues like diet, nutrition, and exercise as well as mental, emotional, and spiritual well-being.

A good example of a holistic practitioner is John C. Pittman, M.D., who works primarily with patients with HIV infection and AIDS. A staunch advocate of bio-oxidative therapies, he created the following "Comprehensive HIV/AIDS Protocol" designed to assist in the healing of many aspects of the patient's being:

1. *Intravenous Ozone:* Start with small amounts at low concentrations and increase gradually as tolerated on a near-daily basis.

2. *Intravenous Hydrogen Peroxide:* A dilute solution is given two to three times a week.

3. *Intravenous Vitamin C:* Seventy grams along with other vitamins, minerals, and antiviral agents is given once or twice a week.

4. *EDTA Chelation:* Using half the standard dose of EDTA, a synthetic amino acid. This involves a series of intravenous infusions containing EDTA and various other substances.

5. *External Oxygenation:* Using devices that spray hot ozonated water, then followed by a bath with a high concentration of hydrogen peroxide.

6. *Hyperbaric Oxygen Chamber:* Used immediately following ozone infusion, whether by rectal insufflation, autohemotherapy, or intravenous application.

7. *Metabolic and Intestinal Detoxification:* Three-day supplemented fast combined with intestinal cleanser and colonic irrigation.

8. *Raw and Living Food Diet:* Including green drinks (such as spirulina and wheat grass juice) to stimulate enzyme pathways.

9. *Nutritional Supplements:* Large quantities of antioxidants, sulfur-containing amino acids, specific immune-stimulating herbs, and hydrochloric acid to improve digestion.

10. *Exercise:* Daily aerobic exercise to elevate heart rate and improve oxygen delivery to tissues.[2]

In the following five chapters, we examine a variety of natural approaches to health that can complement ozone and hydrogen peroxide therapy. Using material from a wide variety of sources—with special emphasis on the work of bio-oxidative therapy practitioners—we examine body cleansing, diet, nutrition, aerobic exercise, and breathing, as well as mental, emotional, and spiritual well-being.

8

BODY CLEANSING

Your body is perfectly designed to be a self-cleaning organism. It eliminates toxins efficiently through exhaling, sneezing, coughing, vomiting, moving the bowels, urinating, sweating, and by occasionally forming boils and pimples. In theory, the body should be able to eliminate all of the waste matter from normal metabolism as well as the toxic matter taken into the body through breathing, eating, and other contact with the environment.

Unfortunately, our modern lifestyles often make it difficult for the body to perform its natural functions efficiently. Lack of exercise, poor diet, overeating, smoking, environmental pollution, pesticides in food, and the stresses of daily life place unnatural burdens on the body, making the efficient elimination of toxins difficult. That is especially true if one is already ill and one's body is further intoxicated by medications, radiation, or chemotherapy.

Hydrogen peroxide and ozone are powerful oxidizers. Although the dozens of studies cited in this book testify to their health-enhancing qualities, bio-oxidative therapies can also cause problems: The accelerated oxidation of viruses, bacteria, fungi, diseased cells, and other substances the body no longer needs can cause a toxic buildup in the body if it is not able to eliminate them efficiently.

Body cleansing can serve two main purposes: First, by helping the body to get rid of its toxic load, it enhances the body's ability to perform its normal functions of elimination more efficiently. Second, it prevents toxic overload, which can lead to discomfort and disease, from occurring. In the following pages we examine several methods of body cleansing. Some can be accomplished easily at home, while others require the guidance or assistance of a qualified health practitioner.

Intestinal Cleansing

Intestinal cleansing is an important complement to bio-oxidative therapies. Physicians like Frank Shallenberger and John C. Pittman insist on intestinal cleansing regimens before they begin to treat AIDS patients with ozone.

Advocates of intestinal cleansing maintain that over many years, toxic matter can accumulate in the colon and the small intestine. Impacted fecal matter and mucoid (defined by Robert Gray as "any slimy, sticky, gluelike substance originating in the body for the purpose of holding substances to be eliminated in suspension,"[1] such as feces) tend to build up and pollute our inner environment through the intestine. Constipation has reached epidemic proportions in industrialized nations, and problems such as diverticulitis and spastic colon, as well as other health problems, may be due to a dirty, congested colon. Difficulty in assimilating nutrients, fatigue, and headaches may also be caused by a buildup of toxins in the intestines.

Dr. Horst Kief believes that when the colon is filled with excrement, the ozone cannot reach all of the pathogenic flora residing in the intestine, especially for the fungi that may have settled in between the intestinal vili and the crypts. For this reason, Dr. Kief recommends a thorough cleansing of the large intestine before ozone is administered through rectal insufflation. Furthermore, Dr. Kief feels that the insufflation properties are enhanced if the bowel cleansing is done with ozonated water.[2]

A number of safe, natural intestinal cleansing methods include ingesting high-fiber psyllium husks or another natural substance such as Kalenite, pectin, or agar, which can be found in any good natural-food store.

Dozens of plants also help naturally loosen, soften, or dissolve impacted stools and mucoid matter in the intestines. According to *The Colon Health Handbook* (see resources), they include aloe, barberry, bayberry bark, grapes, chickweed, goldenseal root, spirulina plankton, and yellow dock root.[3] Many can be taken as teas. It is also possible to buy commercial preparations of a number of herbs that work synergistically to help cleanse the colon. They are found in many health-food stores.

An enema is another natural method of cleansing the colon. There are many types of enemas, including coffee enemas, garlic and chlorophyll enemas, and enemas made of wheat grass juice mixed with water. The idea is to get as much liquid into the higher sections of the colon as possible to receive maximum benefit. Chapters describing enemas are included in a number of books by living-food advocate Ann Wigmore, including *Be Your Own Doctor,* as well as Mark Konlee's *AIDS Control Diet* (see resources). While focusing on AIDS, Konlee's book offers much valuable advice for anyone interested in achieving optimal health through natural means.

Colonic irrigation is a more intensive way to clean the large intestine. This type of cleansing involves circulating water through the colon under light pressure. The colonic debris is then carried out with the water.

A fairly recent development in ozone therapy has been the design of colonic systems using ozonated water. One such system, codesigned by Actual Water Services and Ozone Services in Canada (figure 8.1), utilizes a standard ozone generator and a specialized gravity-based water system. Practitioners and patients alike feel that colonics done with ozonated water are more effective than ordinary tap water. In addition to introducing small amounts of therapeutic ozone into the colon, the water itself is completely free from the pathogens, heavy metals, and chemicals often found in municipal or well water. Disposable materials should always be used with this procedure, which is usually done by a certified colon therapist. Many are members of the American Colon Therapy Association.

While painless and safe, many colon and intestinal cleansing methods can remove "friendly bacteria" from the intestine along with the impacted fecal matter and mucoid. Supplementing one's diet with acidophilus (found in any natural-food store) is recommended to restore a healthy level of intestinal flora.

Juice Therapy

The use of fresh fruit and vegetable juices has been recommended by naturopathic physicians for over sixty years. At the famous Gerson Clinic in Mexico, large amounts of fresh raw juices have been an important component of the holistic cancer protocol for over forty years.[4] Many

Figure 8.1. Ozonated gravity feed colon therapy system. (Reprinted courtesy of Actual Water Services and Yanco Industries Ltd.)

people have also used fresh, natural juices as part of a holistic treatment of AIDS. Bottled or canned juices are considered to be of little value in a body-cleansing regimen, because processing and storage robs them of essential vitamins and enzymes that are important for healing.

In addition to providing concentrated amounts of easily digestible vitamins, minerals, and enzymes, many fruits and vegetables contain medicinal properties. Apples, for example, are mildly laxative, while carrots—in addition to being rich in the antioxidant beta carotene—are natural purifiers and gently cleanse the intestine.

The juices that are most often recommended for intestinal cleansing are fresh carrot juice (either prepared alone or mixed with smaller amounts of celery, spinach, or beets) and fresh apple juice, which can be made with a few added carrots or lettuce leaves. Mark Konlee recommends a juice made of endive, parsley, romaine lettuce, carrot tops, beet greens, and celery for people infected with HIV. One-half cup of cultured cabbage juice three times daily is suggested to heal mucous membranes and help restore the viability of the gastrointestinal tract.[5]

Fruits and vegetables must be carefully washed before they are placed in the juicer. Use organically grown produce whenever possible, because they are free of free-radical-producing chemical pesticides and fertilizers. They often cost a bit more but are worth the extra expense.

It is important that the juices be consumed as soon as possible after they are prepared. If fresh juices are a part of a body-cleansing regimen, drink as much as you comfortably can during the day. A quart or more daily is recommended for people dealing with a serious disease, such as cancer or AIDS. Fortunately, these juices are delicious and are easily tolerated by most people.

Some people partake of a "juice fast" and consume nothing but fresh, raw juices for days at a time; others consume two to three large glasses of fresh juice every day in addition to their regular meals. If you are interested in fresh juices, consider investing in a good, reliable juicer. There are also a number of excellent books on juicing (which contain recipes for a variety of health conditions) in print. A few are listed in the resources section of this book.

Fasting

Therapeutic fasting is an ancient method of body purification that has been popular since biblical times. Although the human organism can live without air for only a few minutes and without water for days, it can go without eating for several months. Fasting—especially when combined with one of the methods of colon cleansing above—can enable the body to discharge years of accumulated toxins.

There are many different types of fasts. Some people ingest nothing but pure water during a fast, while others fast with vegetable broth, herbal teas, or certain fruits alone, such as grapes. Fasts can last from one day to several weeks or more. While a simple juice-only fast of one day is safe for most people, fasting with only water, or for periods longer than one day, should be attempted only under the supervision of a qualified health professional. Light exercise and deep, rhythmic breathing are often recommended with fasts and tend to make the fasting process much easier. As cravings for food often occur when we fast, avoid watching others eat during the fasting period! The famous Swiss naturopath Dr. Alfred Vogel offered the following sound advice on fasting in his book *The Nature Doctor:*

> During the fast it is necessary to maintain the normal rhythm of movement and take adequate rest. All extremes are harmful, so avoid them. For instance, do not spend your days on the couch or in bed in the mistaken belief that you must conserve your energy while not eating. On the other hand, do not engage in arduous sports or walks; it would do you no good. The balance of movement and rest during your fast will revive you, restoring vitality and giving you a new foundation for health and well-being.[6]

Skin Scrubbing

Everyone knows that the skin is our largest organ, but most do not know that it is a primary means by which toxins are eliminated from the body every day, mostly through sweating. Rubbing the skin with a skin scrubber (often a natural sponge known as a *loofah* or a pad made of tightly woven rope) helps stimulate the skin and get rid of dead skin cells. Another good skin scrubber is a brush with bristles made of natural vegetable fibers. The preferred method is to brush the skin with long, even strokes in the direction toward the heart. Avoid brushing the face. Skin brushing is an invigorating experience and can be done gently but firmly. One skin brushing in the morning before your shower and one at bedtime is pleasurable and helps make the skin a more vital organ of elimination.

Dr. Juliane Sacher of Frankfurt offers the following suggestion to aid both in moisturizing the skin and in facilitating the elimination of toxins through the skin: Take one cup of olive oil and heat it until a drop of water will "burst" on contact. Let the oil cool to body temperature and then rub it over the entire body. Wash off the oil and then rest. Although applying olive oil can be a great deal of fun (especially when done with a partner), Dr. Sacher recommends that it be done no more than twice a year.[7]

Saunas and Steam Baths

Healers from around the world have long recommended the therapeutic use of steam baths and saunas. They have been an integral part of a healthy lifestyle among the Russians, Scandinavians, Arabs, and

Figure 8.2. Steam cabinet for use in ozone applications.
(Photo reprinted courtesy of Ozone Services.)

American Indians for hundreds, if not thousands, of years. My grandfather, who was a native of Odessa on the Black Sea, used to go to an old Russian *banya* on Manhattan's Lower East Side at least once a week and found it refreshing, relaxing, and invigorating.

Saunas and steam baths increase body metabolism. They make us sweat and enable the body to release toxins through the skin. They also disperse congestion, increase circulation, and help the immune system fight off diseases by raising body temperature. When combined with pure water, fresh juices, and skin scrubbing techniques, they can be especially effective in body cleansing.

We mentioned before that one of the most pleasant and least invasive ways to use ozone therapy is through the steam-bath method. This method utilizes a specially designed steam cabinet to accommodate an inflow of ozone gas that mixes with the steam. The body absorbs the amount of ozone it needs through the open pores of the skin. Special care is taken so that the subject does not breathe in the ozone gas while enjoying the steam bath: The space for the person's head and neck is padded with towels to avoid leakage and a fan is placed behind the individual to prevent inhalation of gas. A typical bath can last from ten to fifteen minutes at a suggested concentration of 30–40 gamma of ozone (30–40 µg ozone/liter oxygen), which flows continuously through the unit. This method is often used as a spa treatment for healthy people or to supplement other types of biooxidative therapies. A typical steam cabinet costs around $2000 without a generator, but an increasing number of health practitioners are using them in their practices and offer them at nominal cost to patients. One of these steam cabinets is shown in figure 8.2.

As with all body-cleansing techniques, moderation is the key. Do not spend more time in a "hot room" than is comfortable; with practice, you will be able to remain inside for longer periods of time. Although most health clubs maintain high levels of cleanliness in their saunas and steam rooms, some do not. As a result, bacteria and molds tend to multiply. If you are suffering from an immune-related health problem, avoid saunas and steam rooms unless you are certain that they are regularly cleaned and disinfected. People suffering from high blood pressure or heart or circulatory diseases should consult their physician before using a steam room or sauna.

The Experience of Body Cleansing: Not Always Pleasant

Many people judge the process of body cleansing as "dirty" or "wrong." Diarrhea, for example, is an efficient way for the body to quickly free itself from substances that are toxic or irritating. While many of us feel uncomfortable when we experience occasional diarrhea, it is essentially a normal function of a body striving for health.

Many of the techniques mentioned in this chapter may enable the body to experience higher levels of cleansing through discharge. We may notice that our body odor is stronger, our urine may change its characteristic color, and bowel movements may be darker, stronger smelling, and more frequent than we are accustomed to. Some people may even experience nausea, weakness, fever, and headache. While it is useful to monitor these reactions to body cleansing, it is also important to respect the body's process of discharge. By carefully applying the principles of body cleansing described in this chapter, such reactions should be minimal and temporary.

9

AN OXYGENATION DIET

A growing number of bio-oxidative practitioners feel that changes in diet and lifestyle are necessary to complement ozone or hydrogen peroxide treatment and restore long-term health. Although choosing the right foods is a highly personal matter and no one diet is correct for everyone, this chapter explores some of the components to several comprehensive nutritional programs that can complement bio-oxidative therapies for most individuals. From time to time, references will be made to those suffering from specific health problems, such as cancer or AIDS.

Remember that the material provided in this chapter (as in all chapters in this section) is *for information only*. Consult a qualified professional for specific guidance regarding your personal dietary needs. Entire books are devoted to the subject covered in this chapter. If you are interested in learning more about a specific approach to diet and nutrition, consult one or more of the diet books listed in the resources section.

An Oxygenation Diet

What kind of diet are we looking for? Ideally, we want to strive for a dietary program that will satisfy the following needs:

1. It will be low in elements that produce free-radical damage, while being high in those that protect against and destroy free radicals.

2. It will provide adequate amounts of protein, carbohydrates, minerals, and fiber.

3. It will be low in fat, sugar, and salt.

4. It will provide additional oxygen to the body that will help oxygenate tissues and other body cells.

We mentioned earlier that a major source of free radicals is environmental pollutants. Many of those pollutants come from what we eat and drink because of the pesticide residues found in the food supply. According to the *Handbook of Pest Management in Agriculture,* by 1990 the increase in pesticide use in the United States had jumped 3300 percent since 1945.[1]

Unless we own greenhouses and grow only organic fruits and vegetables, it is not easy to avoid pesticides and other pollutants completely. One way is to purchase only organically grown foods, which are free of persistent chemical fertilizers and pesticides. Although they are somewhat more expensive and often unavailable at the local supermarket, many feel that the long-term benefits are well worth the trouble.

The second way to reduce our consumption of pesticides and other free-radical-producing substances in food is to eat as low as possible on the food chain. The food chain refers to the series of living things that are considered to be linked, because each thing feeds upon what is before it in a series. The higher up the food chain we go, the higher levels of pesticide residues we encounter.

For example, when we ingest protein from the flesh or the egg of a chicken that has eaten grain sprayed with pesticides, we are consuming a far greater concentration of pesticides than if we were to consume the protein directly from the grain. Eggs and dairy products generally contain about two-fifths the pesticide residues found in meat; vegetables contain only one-seventh as much. Fruits and legumes contain one-eighth, while grains and cereals have only one-twenty-fourth the pesticide residues found in meat.[2]

Antioxidant Nutrition

Basically, a good oxygenating diet consists of fresh, whole, and oxygen-rich foods that also provide an abundant amount of antioxidants such as beta carotene, vitamin C, and vitamin E. Depending on their nature, these antioxidants will either protect cells from free-radical damage or serve as scavengers to "mop up" excess free radicals in the body.

Beta Carotene

The best sources of beta carotene include fresh carrots, leafy greens, squash (especially yellow squash such as pumpkin), yams, sweet potatoes, and broccoli. The best fruit sources include cantaloupes, apricots, and peaches. One of the best sources of all is nori, a seaweed that is used extensively in Japanese cuisine. Found in health-food stores and oriental groceries, it can easily be added to soups and stews. In her book *Good Health in a Toxic World: The Complete Guide to Fighting Free Radicals*, Sara Shannon recommends four servings of beta carotene–rich foods a day, with additional supplementation as needed.[3] We examine nutritional supplements in detail in the following chapter.

Vitamin C

The best sources of vitamin C include citrus fruits, tomatoes, strawberries, leafy green vegetables, broccoli, Brussels sprouts, green peppers, and acerola berries. Three or more daily servings are recommended from this group, although many bio-oxidative practitioners recommend additional supplementation.

Vitamin E

Cold-pressed and unrefined vegetable oils (such as canola, linseed or flaxseed, olive, safflower, and soy) are very high in vitamin E. Whole grains (including oatmeal and brown rice), dried beans and other legumes, and leafy green vegetables are good sources as well. Sara Shannon recommends a daily intake of three servings of leafy green vegetables, two servings of grains, and two teaspoons of unrefined vegetable oil. As with vitamin C, therapists working with bio-oxidative therapies often recommend extra vitamin E.

B Vitamins

A number of vitamins make up the B vitamin family, including B_1 (thiamin), B_2 (riboflavin), B_3 (niacin), B_6 (pyridoxine), folacin (folic acid), and B_{12} (cyanocobalamin). Together, they are known as the vitamin B complex. The B vitamins are necessary to aid in the proper digestion and the efficient utilization of carbohydrates, and they help break down proteins so they can be efficiently used by the body. They also aid body growth and help keep the nervous system in optimal condition, which is important in immunoregulation. The vitamin B complex has also been found to be an antioxidant cofactor, which means that the B vitamins play a supportive role in enabling the antioxidants listed above to work more effectively.

B vitamins are found primarily in grains, dried beans and peas, and seeds and nuts, especially oats, wheat germ, and peanuts. They are also found in brewer's yeast, a highly nutritious product available at many natural-food stores. A varied diet using these foods will help to preserve good health and can complement most bio-oxidative treatment programs.

There are a number of other antioxidant cofactors, including the minerals selenium and zinc, as well as the amino acid glutathione. Since many people have deficiencies in these substances, we discuss them in the following chapter on vitamin and mineral supplements.

A New Basic Four

In 1956, the famous Four Basic Food Groups model was created by the United States Department of Agriculture, which set the standards for a healthy diet for Americans. Developed under the influence of the meat and dairy interests, it emphasized a high consumption of meat, eggs, and dairy products, which made up half of the four groups. As consumers became more aware of the serious dangers of high-cholesterol and high-fat diets that resulted from following the Four Food Groups plan, it was replaced by Dietary Guidance for Americans in 1990, which expanded the four food groups to five. However, that plan was also influenced by the meat and dairy interests and still placed strong emphasis on an animal-based diet. It was replaced the following year by the Food Pyramid, which places somewhat stronger emphasis on plant foods. Although the Food Pyramid represents an important departure from past recommendations, many progressive nutritionists feel that it does not go far enough.

A dietary plan that is most likely to complement the benefits of bio-oxidative therapies is the little-known New Four Food Groups created by the Physicians Committee for Responsible Medicine (PCRM) in Washington, D.C. First proposed in 1991, it is seen as an "optimal diet" that not only provides adequate nutrition but can actually help prevent many diet-related diseases, such as hypertension, cancer, and atherosclerosis. Like the original four groups, they are easy to remember, but they emphasize plant foods rather than foods of animal origin. This plan features four primary food groups, with "optional" foods to be eaten sparingly.[4]

Group I: Whole Grains

This group includes bread, pasta, hot and cold cereal, rice, millet, barley, bulgur, buckwheat, groats, and tortillas. These foods provide complex carbohydrates, protein, B vitamins, and zinc.

Five or more servings are recommended daily from this group. A serving is considered to be one-half cup of cooked cereal, one ounce of dry cereal, or one slice of bread.

Group II: Vegetables

Group II includes dark green leafy vegetables like collards, kale, mustard and turnip greens, and cruciferous vegetables, which include broccoli, cabbages, Brussels sprouts, and cauliflower. These vegetables are good sources of a variety of vitamins (especially vitamin C and riboflavin), minerals (particularly calcium and iron), and dietary fiber, often lacking in standard diets. Dark yellow vegetables (including carrots, squash, sweet potatoes, and pumpkin) are also excellent sources of beta carotene.

Three or more daily servings (one cup raw or one-half cup cooked) from this group are recommended.

Group III: Legumes

Dried peas, beans, chickpeas, and lentils are good sources of protein, dietary fiber, iron, calcium, zinc, and B vitamins. Foods in this category also include textured soy protein, soy milk, tofu (soybean curd), and tempeh, made from fermented soybeans. Two to three daily servings (one-half cup of cooked beans, four ounces of tofu or tempeh, or eight ounces of soy milk) from this group are recommended.

Group IV: Fruits

All fruits are recommended by the PCRM, to be eaten as close to their natural state as possible. Of special interest are citrus fruits, tomatoes (technically a fruit), and strawberries (which are all good sources of vitamin C), as well as cantaloupes and apricots, which are high in beta carotene.

A minimum of three servings daily from this group is recommended. One medium piece of fruit, one-half cup of cooked fruit, or one-half cup of fresh fruit juice constitutes a serving.

Optional Foods

To the chagrin of the meat and dairy industries, the Physicians Committee for Responsible Medicine placed meat, fish, and dairy products (along with nuts, seeds, and oils) into the Optional Foods group to be used as condiments. While they are not banned, the committee felt that they should no longer serve as the focal point for the optimal American diet, as they have in the past. PCRM Chairperson Neal Bernard, M.D., called this plan "a modest proposal" that if adopted could have a profound impact on America's high incidence of heart disease and cancer. For more information about this organization, consult the resources section of this book.

What the Bio-oxidative Healers Suggest

A number of prominent individuals who have worked with bio-oxidative therapies (and patients who have undergone those therapies) have offered sound dietary guidance as adjuncts to the therapeutic use of medical ozone and hydrogen peroxide. We do not advocate any particular diet but think several are worthy of consideration. They complement each other extensively.

In his monograph *Workbook on Free Radical Chemistry and Hydrogen Peroxide Metabolism*, Dr. Charles H. Farr confines his dietary advice to the following suggestions:

> Patients should be counseled to limit dietary fats and oils (all types) to approximately 20 to 25% of their total caloric intake. They should especially avoid heated, extracted and refined fats which are rich in lipid peroxide precursors of free radicals. Refined carbohydrates and simple sugars should be avoided and substituted with unrefined, complex starches

containing adequate dietary fiber, obtained from whole grains, vegetables and whole fruit.[5]

In his book *The Oxygen Breakthrough*, Sheldon Saul Hendler, M.D., recommends an "ideal" diet to his patients that is very much in harmony with both the New Four and Dr. Farr's recommendations. Dr. Hendler's "high-oxygen diet" includes the following:

- no more than 100 milligrams of cholesterol daily
- no more than 20 percent fat, with increased amounts of polyunsaturates and monosaturates and decreased amounts of saturates
- at least 65 percent carbohydrates, with emphasis on complex, unrefined carbohydrates
- 12 to 15 percent protein, with increased reliance on vegetable protein
- 50 to 60 grams of dietary fiber[6]

At the Hospital Santa Monica in Mexico, Dr. Kurt Donsbach offers the following modest food recommendations (along with friendly practical advice) to help patients achieve a higher level of health and well-being both at the hospital and after they return home.

1. Do eat a bowl of oatmeal or other whole grain cereal every morning. (We shouldn't have to tell you to avoid white sugar and white flour products as much as possible.)

2. Do eat four cupfuls of vegetables daily—half raw and half cooked. It will surprise you how many vegetables really exist. Try them all.

3. Do eat one cupful of fruit daily, preferably raw unless unavailable.

4. Do eat only the following fats: butter, olive oil, peanut oil. *Margarine and unsaturated oils are the worst foods you can put into your body.* (Flaxseed oil, bottled in black and kept refrigerated, is the only exception—it can be used therapeutically at one tablespoon once or twice daily.)

5. Do reduce coffee consumption to one cup daily. Get in the herb tea habit.

6. Do eat your heaviest meals at breakfast and lunch [and have your] light meal at night. This is the hardest rule to follow for most people.

7. Do eat a minimum of five servings of chicken, fish or turkey each week. You can have a serving of beef or pork occasionally. If you are a vegetarian by choice, eat seeds and nuts to supplement your diet. Eggs and dairy products may be used as desired.

8. Do not combine fruits or fruit juices with concentrated proteins (meats, dairy products, eggs). This will produce gas and discomfort.

9. Do eat whole grains, freshly baked breads and rolls.

10. Do use a seasoning salt made up of potassium, sodium, calcium, magnesium, lysine and kelp as your flavor enhancer.

11. Be positive and happy when you eat. Your digestive system will work better.[7]

The AIDS Control Diet

The sixth edition of *The AIDS Control Diet* lists a number of "foods that heal."[8] Although they are intended primarily for people infected with HIV, these foods are good for anyone who is involved in the healing process unless prohibited by a physician. Many people fear that a health-oriented diet is limited, but, as we will see in the following diet plans, that need not be the case.

Vegetables

All vegetables are allowed on the AIDS Control Diet except iceberg lettuce, while cucumbers and tomatoes are to be eaten sparingly. The vegetables in *italic* type should be eaten raw; many of them can be made into salads or fresh juices.

Sprouts (including *wheat grass, red clover*, radish, and alfalfa), artichokes, *asparagus*, avocado, *bamboo shoots*, banana pepper, *endive*, escarole, *parsley*, Boston lettuce, *dandelion greens, beet greens, beets*, soy bean sprouts, *cabbage*, collard greens, bok choy, *broccoli*, cauliflower, Chinese cabbage, kale, kohlrabi, *carrots*, celery, eggplant, *garlic, onions, jalapeño pepper*, lamb's quarters, *leeks*, okra, olives, potatoes, sweet potatoes, rutabagas, turnips, *green peas, green beans, pumpkin, radish*, red sweet pepper, sea kale, shallot, *spinach*, squash, *Swiss chard*, and *turnip greens*. Sauerkraut is also recommended.

The best carbohydrate sources include boiled potatoes, rutabagas, turnips, and squash, while carrots and beets are best eaten raw.

High-Protein Sources

Gelatine (animal or vegetable); soy milk blended with fresh pineapple, kiwi or papaya, and/or lemon juice; split pea soup; lentil soup; vegetarian chili; almond milk; pumpkin seed milk; and plain yogurt. Ten grams or more of dried brewer's yeast, barley grass juice, or wheat grass juice is recommended as a supplement. Creamed cottage cheese, bean soup, cooked lima beans, canned sardines, and canned salmon can be used in moderation.

Fats and Oils That Heal

Olive oil and butter. One to two tablespoons of flaxseed oil can be mixed with potatoes and salads.

Seasonings

Paprika, crushed red pepper, apple cider vinegar, and thyme, as well as natural commercial seasoning mixtures like Spike. Sea salt and black pepper can be used in moderation.

Gluten-Free Grains

Rice (white or brown), rye crisp crackers, and products made with corn, quinoa, amaranth, buckwheat, millet, spelt, kamut, or other gluten-free grains.

Fruit

Raw lemons, limes, grapefruit, kiwi fruit, papaya, pineapple, and unsweetened applesauce are recommended in unlimited quantities, while a maximum of one daily serving of all other fruits is suggested.

Sweeteners

Raw, unfiltered honey; sucanat; raw cane sugar; brown sugar; date sugar; and blackstrap molasses are to be used in moderation.

Beverages

Filtered water, spring water, and mineral water are recommended over unfiltered municipal water. Herbal teas such as rose hip tea are recommended between meals. Green tea (available in oriental markets) is an excellent health-giving tea with antioxidant properties.

The Raw Food and Living Food Diet

The late Ann Wigmore, D.D., N.D., was well known in the holistic community for her radical approach to helping people heal themselves of cancer, heart disease, Candida, diabetes, AIDS, and other "incurable" diseases through eating plant foods low on the food chain. Believing that raw, uncooked, fermented, and sprouted foods are easily digested, are free of chemical additives, and contain a minimum of pesticides (since they are low on the food chain), "Dr. Ann's" living-food diet includes fresh fruits and vegetables, seeds, grains, and nuts. Methods of preparation include juicing, sprouting, fermenting, and light blending. She believes that foods prepared in those ways allow the body's cells to fully absorb the life force produced by the enzymes of live foods, many of which, coincidentally, contain hydrogen peroxide. Many living foods can be grown indoors as greens and as sprouts.

In her book *Overcoming AIDS* (see resources), Wigmore lists what she calls "the most important foods for total health":

Greens: Sunflower, cabbage, buckwheat, dandelion, watercress, parsley, lamb's quarters.

Top of the ground vegetables: Corn, red pepper, celery, radish, zucchini, summer squash, mushrooms.

Fermented foods: Cauliflower, beets, carrots, seed cheese, rejuvelac (a drink made by adding water to sprouted wheat seeds, which, after several days, can be poured off and consumed).

Fruits: Watermelon, peeled apples, peaches, figs, dates, avocado, tomato, bananas.

Grains: Rye, millet, corn, wheat.

Protein: Almonds, pine nuts, sunflower seeds.

Sprouts: Alfalfa, fenugreek, mung bean, radish.

Seaweed: Dulse.[9]

Ann Wigmore's approach is a radical departure from the standard American diet, in which animal products, processed foods, cooked foods, sugar, and salt are consumed in excessive amounts. Although her diet is admittedly unconventional, many holistic healers believe that it is probably the best one to follow if one wants to make major changes in one's life as part of the healing process: Live more simply, free the body of toxins, enhance the body's natural healing powers, and consume only the purest and freshest of foods. While some may feel that a total raw-food diet is too extreme, certain aspects of this diet can easily become integrated into one's personal diet plan. Two of Ann Wigmore's books (which include many recipes), as well as the address of her healing center, are included in the resources section of this book.

10

Nutritional Supplements and Healing Herbs

In an ideal world, food supplementation would not be necessary. We would be so in touch with our bodies that we would instinctively know what we need to eat in what amounts. Our foods would be organically grown under ideal climatic conditions, picked from the garden or orchard not far from home, and eaten in their natural state within a few hours or days of harvesting.

Reality is different. For the most part, we often have no idea what we should eat, let alone how much. Nearly all of our produce is harvested weeks before it is ripe, often transported over long distances (sometimes from around the world), and subjected to days or weeks of storage. Many of our canned and packaged foods have essential vitamins, minerals, and enzymes refined out of them during processing. By the time they arrive at the dinner table, many of the foods we eat have far less nutrition than they originally contained. For that reason, a growing number of nutritionists are recommending food supplements to provide a "safety net" in order to avoid vitamin and mineral deficiencies and the diseases they can cause.

While the bio-oxidative diets described in the previous chapter (along with broad-spectrum daily multivitamin and mineral supplements containing ingredients with antioxidant activity) are designed to provide adequate nutrition under normal circumstances, people who are challenged by ill health often require additional elements that will help strengthen the immune system and optimize the benefits of bio-oxidative therapies.

This chapter is not a course in nutrition. Its purpose is to introduce and discuss some of the food supplements and herbs that are often used to enhance the benefits of bio-oxidative therapies. While some references are from mainstream nutritional publications, I also draw on the clinical experience of leading dietitians, physicians, and other practitioners who work with the nutritional aspects of healing. It is hoped that this chapter will inspire you to gain a more complete understanding of the role of vitamins and minerals in the healing process. In addition, a number of books that provide more extensive information are listed in the resources section.

While supplements can be useful as daily additions to a good diet, they are often not recommended to be taken within several hours of the time that one undergoes bio-oxidative therapy—especially intravenous hydrogen peroxide—unless recommended by a physician. It is also important to remember that more is not always better. An excess of certain vitamins and minerals can actually depress immune function.

In the context of this book, a primary goal of food supplementation is to provide adequate amounts of antioxidants to help scavenge excess free radicals and protect other cells from free-radical damage. The three most important elements are beta carotene, vitamin C, and vitamin E. For maximum benefit, it is important to take these antioxidants together, because they produce synergistic effects; they work more effectively as a group than when they are taken alone.

As a general reference, table 10.1 lists the current Reference Daily Intakes (formerly known as Recommended Daily Allowances) for the major vitamins and minerals as determined by the United States Food and Drug Administration and the National Research Council. These estimates, which change from time to time, are based on the amount of nutrients necessary to prevent nutritional deficiencies in both children and adults. Many critics feel that the RDIs are far too low to help people achieve optimal health and should be used more as a guidepost for minimal nutrition than as a nutritional ideal.

Beta Carotene

Beta carotene is a precursor to vitamin A, which means that it must exist before vitamin A is formed. It promotes growth and wound healing and prevents night blindness and diseases of the eye. It is also important for healthy skin and bones and helps maintain the well-being of the

---

Table 10.1. U.S. Reference Daily Intakes for Adults and Children Four Years and Older

Vitamin A	5,000 I.U.
Vitamin C	60 mg
Thiamin (vitamin B_1)	1.5 mg
Riboflavin (vitamin B_2)	1.7 mg
Niacin (vitamin B_3)	20 mg
Pyridoxine (vitamin B_6)	2 mg
Cyanocobalamin (vitamin B_{12})	6 mμg
Folic acid (folacin)	400 μg
Vitamin D	400 I.U.
Vitamin E	30 I.U.
Phosphorous	1 g
Calcium	1 g
Iron	18 mg
Iodine	150 μg
Magnesium	400 mg
Zinc.	15 mg
Copper	2 mg
Biotin.	300 μg
Pantothenic acid	10 mg

Source: U. S. Food and Drug Administration, Code of Federal Regulation 101.9, 1973.

Note: I.U., International Units; g, gram; mg, milligram (1/1000 of a gram); μg, microgram (1/1000 of a milligram).

---

respiratory tract, the throat, and the bronchial region. It is found mostly in all yellow and green vegetables, especially squash, carrots, and sweet potatoes, as well as apricots and cantaloupes.

For a normal adult weighing 70 kg (154 pounds), the DI as determined by the United States Food and Drug Administration is 5000 International Units (I.U.) of vitamin A, or 3 mg of beta carotene. As part of a healing program, between 5000 and 10,000 I.U. (6 mg) is recommended daily. Higher therapeutic amounts may be toxic to some individuals and should be taken only under a physician's supervision.

Vitamin C

Vitamin C is important in helping maintain healthy teeth and gums. It also supports the immune system and is viewed as a major factor in preventing colds. Vitamin C is responsible for the health and maintenance of collagen in the teeth, bones, skin, capillaries, and connective tissue and aids in detoxifying the body of poisons. Known as the "protector vitamin," vitamin C plays an essential role in protecting cells and preventing tissue damage from free radicals. For this reason, some feel that it helps prevent diseases associated with free-radical damage, including heart disease and cancer. In addition to acerola berries, vitamin C is found in citrus fruits and many green vegetables.

The Reference Daily Intake is 60 mg, which many practitioners believe is inadequate. To protect the body from free-radical damage, a maintenance dose of 1000 mg (1 gram) of vitamin C is often recommended, while 1 to 3 grams per day is suggested for those with a serious disease like cancer or AIDS. Some physicians recommend even more. Dr. John C. Pittman's comprehensive HIV/AIDS protocol includes 70 grams of intravenous vitamin C (along with other vitamins, minerals, and antiviral agents) once or twice a week.[1]

Vitamin E

Because vitamin E promotes circulation and helps prevent blood clots, it has gotten much publicity for its role in helping to reduce the risk of heart disease. It is also important for the healing of wounds, burns, scars, and other skin problems and helps protect the body's store of vitamins A and D. As a powerful antioxidant, vitamin E is a scavenger of free radicals. It is found primarily in vegetable oils, wheat germ, green leafy vegetables, eggs, and butter.

The RDI for vitamin E is 30 I.U. However, many holistic practitioners who work with bio-oxidative therapies and progressive heart specialists who believe that vitamin E can reduce the risk of heart attack recommend 400–800 I.U. daily.

Vitamin B$_6$

Vitamin B$_6$, or pyridoxine, is called an antioxidant cofactor because it synergizes with vitamins C and E and helps them work more effectively.

This vitamin plays an important role in converting fats, proteins, and carbohydrates into usable energy. It also is of importance to the thymus gland, which plays a major role in immunoregulation. The primary sources of vitamin B_6 include wheat germ, brewer's yeast, whole grains, peanuts, bananas, and cabbage.

The RDI for this vitamin is only 2 mg, although many believe that 25 mg or more a day is valuable for people who are dealing with a health problem. Dr. Juliane Sacher recommends 20–60 mg a day for her AIDS/HIV-positive patients (her complete vitamin and mineral supplement protocol is included in table 10.2).

Nutritionists point out that all members of the B group of vitamins should be taken in proportionate amounts. For that reason, any supplements of vitamin B_6 can be taken as part of a general multivitamin or B-complex formula.

Coenzyme Q_{10}

Coenzyme Q_{10} is not a vitamin but an energy coenzyme that is essential for the production of adenosine triphosphate (ATP), or cellular energy. Coenzyme Q_{10} has been the subject of much research. As an important antioxidant, it works with vitamin E to scavenge free radicals. It is often recommended for people challenged by diseases like AIDS and chronic fatigue, as well as to help slow the aging process.

Coenzyme Q_{10} is normally synthesized by the body, but it is believed that as people approach middle age, production of this coenzyme slows down. While there is no RDI for this substance, a daily supplement of 10–30 mg is considered adequate.

Selenium

Selenium is one of those "miracle" minerals believed to protect us from cancer, counteract heavy metal toxicity, and slow the aging process. An antioxidant and free-radical scavenger, selenium synergizes with vitamin E in the body to mop up free radicals more effectively. Dr. Hendler notes that selenium "appears to influence favorably *every* component of the immune system."[2]

This mineral is found primarily in seafood, meat, and vegetables, but its presence varies widely in soil. While no RDI has been established for

---

Table 10.2 *Sacher Clinic Daily Nutritional Supplement Recommendations for People with HIV/AIDS*

Vitamin A .... 5,000–10,000 I.U.

Beta carotene.. 25–100 mg

Vitamin C .... 1–3 g

Vitamin E .... 400–1,200 I.U.

Vitamin B_6 .... 0–60 mg

Vitamin B_{12} .... 25–100 μg

Folic acid.. 5–15 mg

Selenium .... 100–200 μg

Magnesium. .... 500–2,000 mg

Calcium... 500–2,000 mg

Potassium aspartate .... 500–1,200 mg

Zinc aspartate .... 50–100 mg

Copper gluconate .... 200–600 μg

N–Acetyl–L–Cystine (an antioxidant) .... 300–1,200 mg

Dr. Sacher also recommends 1–2 tablets daily of ferrum phosphoricum D_6, which is a special type of iron available commercially in trace amounts, like many homeopathic remedies. She suggests that whenever iron is taken, antioxidants should be consumed as well.

Source: Vitamine, Mineralien und Spurenelemente bei HIV-Positiven und AIDS-Patienten *(Frankfurt: Sacher Clinic, 1993). (Reprinted courtesy of Dr. Juliane Sacher.)*

---

selenium, maintenance and protective doses of 50–200 μg are recommended. Excessive amounts of selenium can be toxic.

Zinc

Zinc is another important antioxidant mineral. It is essential for protein synthesis, RNA and DNA formation, carbon dioxide removal, and wound healing. It also promotes and maintains cell membrane fluidity, which helps cell membranes become more receptive to oxygen. Like vitamin B_6, zinc is needed by the thymus gland to manufacture T-cells, so it is considered an important immune booster. That is one reason many people take extra zinc supplements along with vitamin C when they feel a cold coming on.

Zinc is found primarily in whole grains, liver, seafood, sea vegetables, nuts, and carrots. The RDI for zinc is 15 mg, but holistic practitioners recommend 50 mg daily (220 mg of zinc sulfate will provide 50 mg of elemental zinc) for those challenged by disease or who wish to maintain their immune systems at a higher level of efficiency. Dr. Sacher recommends that zinc be taken in proportionate amounts with copper to achieve maximum benefit from both minerals.

Healing Herbs

Several medicinal herbs have been used to complement bio-oxidative therapies. While some are antioxidants, others strengthen the immune system and kill bacteria, viruses, and fungi. The herbs we include here are all easy to use and should not cause adverse side effects of any kind.

Astragalus

Astragalus is an ancient Chinese medicinal herb. The dried root can be made into an important immune-strengthening tonic and has often been prescribed for diarrhea and general fatigue. Astragalus is found through herb catalogs and at oriental herb stores. It can be used as a tea or added (whole) while cooking soups and stews. Astragalus should not be eaten but is removed from the soup as you would remove bay leaves.

Echinacea

Echinacea (coneflower) root is known for its immune-enhancing qualities. Long popular among Native American healers, echinacea has been used to treat microbial and viral infections. Like vitamin C and zinc, it is often recommended to counteract colds and flu. Echinacea is used by people infected with HIV to help strengthen their immune systems. Available in many health-food stores in capsule form and as a tincture, it can be added to water or juice. Echinacea root may also be prepared as a healing tea.

Garlic

Garlic has been used throughout Europe and Asia as a medicinal plant for centuries. In addition to containing a variety of essential vitamins and minerals, garlic is an important immune system strengthener. It acts on bacteria, viruses, and intestinal parasites and can be used as a preventive for many digestive and respiratory conditions. Garlic is also believed to lower cholesterol and blood pressure and raise the level of high-density lipoproteins, which help guard against cardiovascular disease.

Many people make garlic an important part of their daily diets. For those who are not fond of garlic's taste (let alone the aroma it can leave on the breath), powdered garlic supplements in capsule form—especially those made from an aged garlic extract like Kyolic—are recommended instead.

Ginkgo biloba

Ginkgo biloba is the oldest surviving tree species in the world. The leaves have been used by traditional Chinese herbalists to treat heart disease, circulatory problems, and lung disease for thousands of years. Recently ginkgo has become the subject of laboratory and clinical research in the West. An antioxidant, it has been found to lower cholesterol, relieve arthritis, and treat gastrointestinal ulcers. It also may play a role in relieving the symptoms of Alzheimer's disease. Ginkgo biloba extract is available in tablet or tincture form in many health-food stores and in Chinese herbal pharmacies.

Green tea

Green tea has long been a popular health drink in China, Korea, and Japan. It has recently attracted much media attention as an antioxidant with the ability to help lower blood pressure and reduce the risk of cancer and heart disease. Green tea, which contains caffeine, is available in any store that specializes in oriental foods. Health-minded Chinese always drink at least one cup a day of this delicious tea, which is available in different forms and different grades.

Pau d'arco

Pau d'arco comes from the inner bark of a tree found in Brazil. It has antimicrobial, antiviral, and antibacterial properties. Used mostly as a tea, it is said to help strengthen the immune system. It is available in many health-food stores.

11

AEROBIC EXERCISE AND
BREATHING

Oxygen is our source of life. The more oxygen we are able to enjoy, the more we can partake of life itself. Unfortunately, many of us do not breathe to full capacity, and we utilize only a fraction of the life- giving oxygen that we need for the life processes of oxygenation and oxidation.

While bio-oxidative therapies like ozone and hydrogen peroxide can do much to increase these important processes, we can enhance their effectiveness. This chapter examines two very important ways to increase the amount of oxygen available to our bodies so that life can be experienced to the fullest: aerobic exercise and deep, rhythmic breathing.

Aerobic Exercise

Aerobic exercise provides increased oxygenation to the entire body and can be an important adjunct to bio-oxidative therapies. The term *aerobic* simply means "taking place in the presence of oxygen," and aerobic exercise is any form of exercise that increases the amount of oxygen in the body, thereby strengthening the heart and lungs.

Years ago, exercise was rarely recommended for people who were sick. Patients with asthma, heart trouble, or cancer were advised to avoid physical exertion and rest as much as possible. While this may be appropriate for some individuals, a growing number of physicians have learned that most patients *can* participate safely in a wide variety of physical activities, including aerobic exercises, and that it is vital for good health.

Aerobic exercises encompass a wide range of activities from light exertion to major physical challenge: walking, swimming, jogging, inline and ice skating, running, doing calisthenics, dancing, cycling, cross-country skiing, hiking, playing tennis, and practicing martial arts, including t'ai chi, aikido, karate, and boxing. Aerobics can also include specific exercise routines (popularly known simply as "aerobics") and using exercise devices like stair climbers, "rebounder" trampolines, cross-country skiing devices, treadmills, rowing machines, and stationary bicycles. One of the most positive aspects of aerobic exercises is that they can be tailored to our physical condition and exercise goals: We can begin them slowly and then gradually build up to a workout that increases our heartbeat and breathing rate.

Aerobic exercise can provide a number of important physical and psychological benefits. These benefits are synergistic, which means that they work together to provide optimum benefits.

Oxygenation

Through regular moderate aerobic exercise, the heart and circulatory system deliver increased amounts of oxygen to the entire body. This increases both the amount of oxygen and the ATP or life energy delivered to all body cells. It also aids in the process of oxidation, which destroys cells that are sick and weak, replacing them with stronger and healthier cells. When our blood is oxygenated, we feel stronger, healthier, and more alive. We feel more able to perform our tasks and confront the challenges that present themselves in our daily lives with greater resilience and sense of purpose.

Cardiovascular Fitness

Aerobic exercise also strengthens the heart and enables it to provide a reserve capacity of endurance when extra demands are placed on the body. This is especially important if we have been challenged by illness. It also helps us recover our energy faster after physical or emotional burdens are placed on us.

Flexibility

Our bodies are designed to *move,* and regular aerobic exercise helps us achieve a full range of body motion. Because physical exercise (especially swimming and calisthenics) naturally causes us to move all of our joints, our joints will become more flexible, even if they weren't exercised much before. This not only enables us to use our bodies to the fullest, but it decreases the chances of pulling or spraining muscles. When used in conjunction with deep breathing, regular aerobic exercise can also release tension in the chest, neck, and shoulders.

Strength and Endurance

Regular aerobic exercise helps build up our chest muscles and enables us to breathe easier. It also brings about greater overall strength and endurance. We are more able to accomplish our daily tasks and often find we can enjoy activities we couldn't before. My eighty-three-year-old aunt is one such example. Years ago, she didn't have the endurance to join her grandchildren when they hiked on a particular nature trail overlooking the Pacific Ocean. After going through two angioplasties to open up her arteries (and the threat of a coronary bypass operation if the second one didn't work), she decided to change her diet and take a walk every morning and every night near her home. After a year of brisk walking for two hours a day around the neighborhood, she discovered that she was able to join her family on that trail again for the first time in fifteen years.

A Positive Mental Attitude

As we will see in the next chapter, state of mind can have a profound impact on physical well-being. As part of a synergistic "benign cycle," aerobic exercise not only is good for the physical body, but affects our minds as well. Moderate aerobic exercise helps us develop greater self-esteem, optimism, and the feeling that we are able to accomplish what we want to do. It also helps develop a better self-image. After several weeks or months of regular aerobic exercise, we notice that we begin to look better: Excess body fat tends to melt away, our posture improves, our complexion becomes clearer and healthier looking, our eyes become brighter. We also find that different muscle groups gradually develop, sometimes in places we never dreamed possible. Fitness and improved physique help us to feel better about ourselves. This is especially important for people who are dealing with illness: Regular aerobic exercise helps us move away from the image of being sick toward a self-image of attractiveness, health, and vitality.

Before You Exercise

Before you begin an aerobic exercise program, a complete fitness assessment is essential, especially if you have a history of heart disease or high blood pressure or are undergoing medical treatment. The assessment should include an electrocardiogram, a treadmill test, and other tests to determine lung function, strength, and flexibility. Even if you are enjoying good health, it is always a good idea to consult with your physician before undertaking any exercise program.

Proper warm-up before exercise is also important. After fine minutes of light aerobic exercise, many people do stretching exercises, which warm up the muscles gradually and help prepare the body for more strenuous exercise. When your exercise session is complete, a cooling-down period of stretching for several minutes is also recommended.

Keep in Mind . . .

In the context of bio-oxidative therapies, two additional cautions are worth noting: environmental pollution and exercising to excess. The essential idea behind aerobic exercise is to oxygenate the blood in order to achieve a higher level of health and well-being. For many people, jogging or running is the favorite aerobic exercise. Unfortunately, when we run or jog in a polluted environment, such as along city streets jammed with traffic, that type of exercise can be dangerous. As we breathe more frequently, fully, and deeply, we take in increased amounts of environmental pollutants (including ozone, which is generally harmful when taken into the lungs), which increase the number of free radicals in our bodies. In *The Oxygen Breakthrough*, Dr. Hendler cites a number of cases of runners suffering from a variety of health problems because they run in polluted areas.

Dr. Hendler also speaks about the dangers of excessive aerobic exercise. In his book, he cites cases of individuals—often marathon runners and triathlon athletes—who felt guilty unless they ran for hours each day, or who believed in exercising to the point of exhaustion. Many of them became his patients because excess aerobic exercise depressed their immune systems (especially the production of antibodies and natural killer cells) and opened the door to health problems, including chronic fatigue syndrome, asthma, intestinal bleeding, allergies, and respiratory infections.[1]

Moderation: The Key

Moderate exercise on a regular basis is the ideal. Studies have found that weekend athletes who rarely exercise regularly tend to increase the number of free radicals in their bodies, while those who exercise regularly are able to easily get rid of them. In addition, by avoiding over exertion, we tend to enjoy exercising, so we are more likely to want to continue doing it.

Another problem when we begin an exercise program is an "all or nothing" attitude. Many of us feel that if we cannot run a mile, we shouldn't run at all. That makes exercise unpleasant and has sabotaged many a program. Again, moderation is important, especially when we begin. Instead of running for a mile, make your run a half mile. If you don't feel like running, take a brisk walk instead. Rather than spend thirty minutes on the stationary bicycle at full throttle, you can ride at half speed for the half hour or at a faster pace for fifteen minutes. You can gradually build up to faster speeds and longer distances. Exercise instructors often suggest that it is best to begin an exercise regimen slowly and build up the level of activity about 10 percent a week. They also suggest the importance of pacing ourselves: When we are on the running track, we can run for a while and then walk briskly. Or we can rest frequently during the exercise period when we feel we need it. As we gradually build up our strength and endurance, we are better able to participate in longer periods of physical activity.

Exercise Should Be a Pleasure

In general, it is important to grow to like exercise, because if we enjoy what we are doing, we are more likely to continue. Therefore, we should choose an activity that we enjoy. We also can enhance our enjoyment of exercise by choosing the right time or situation. For example, if you get lonely walking alone, do it with friends. If you don't like to walk outdoors, walk at the mall. Over the past few years, I have used a cross-country skiing machine at my office. Sometimes I find it gets boring, so I play music, listen to a recorded book, or watch television while I exercise. Not only do I fulfill my need for exercise, I catch up on the morning news or enjoy a new detective story.

How Much Exercise?

Many physicians recommend at least thirty minutes of exercise several days a week, although thirty minutes may be too long for people beginning an exercise program or who are going through a period of healing. Ask your physician or exercise instructor how you can build up your exercise level gradually and safely.

Breathing

Although all of us breathe, we are often not aware of the quality of our breathing. We tend to take partial, shallow breaths using only the upper part of the lungs, or we often hold our breath (especially when we are tense or nervous) without being conscious of it. When this type of breathing becomes habitual or chronic, we limit the amount of air that we take into our body, which impairs our body's ability to oxygenate the blood and other vital tissues.

Deep, rhythmic breathing is essential for proper oxygenation, and learning how to breathe in a way that involves both the upper and lower parts of the lungs has been viewed as vital by yogis for centuries. Perhaps the most important breath to learn is known as The Yogi Complete Breath first introduced to the West by Yogi Ramacharaka in the early part of this century. In his classic work *The Science of Breath,* he describes performing this breath as follows:

> Stand or sit erect. Breathing through the nostrils, inhale steadily, first filling the lower part of the lungs, which is accompanied by bringing into play the diaphragm, while [distending] exerts a gentle pressure on the abdominal organs, pushing forward the front walls of the abdomen. Then fill the middle part of the lungs, pushing out the lower ribs, breastbone and chest. Then fill the higher portion of the lungs, protruding the upper chest, thus lifting the chest, including the upper six or seven pairs of ribs. In the final movement, the lower part of the abdomen will be slightly drawn in, which movement gives the lungs a support and also helps to fill the highest part of the lungs.

Yogi Ramacharaka reminds us that this breath does not consist of three distinct movements, but is one continuous, fluid movement. He recommends that we retain this breath for a couple of seconds and then exhale slowly, drawing in the abdomen slightly as the air leaves the lungs. He recommends that we relax the chest and abdomen after the air is released.[2]

The Yogi Complete Breath can be done whenever we feel like it. Although at first we may want to do this breath during a period of quiet contemplation or just before we begin our exercise program, gradually we can begin consciously breathing fully and deeply in more and more of our daily activities, until deep, rhythmic breathing becomes a normal part of our lives. In addition to Yogi Ramacharaka's classic work, many other books about yoga offer instruction on deep, rhythmic breathing. Some, like *The Oxygen Breakthrough* mentioned before, offer a number of easy-to-follow breathing exercises.

Only living people breathe; dead people don't. The more we breathe, the more alive we are. And the more we practice deep, rhythmic breathing either alone or in conjunction with aerobic exercise, the more we partake of oxygen: the essence of life itself.

12

EMOTIONS, MIND, AND SPIRIT

Donald M. Epstein, D.C., the principal author of *The Twelve Stages of Healing,* has often said that healing is "an inside job." He means that the most essential components to healing, such as life force, harmony, regeneration, and repair are not given to us by others but come from within. Innate healing power is part of our birthright and is within reach of every one of us. In his essay "There Is No Cure for Healing," Dr. Epstein writes:

> Healing is a process, not a magical event. Nothing new is added to your body or mind. . . . Nothing is taken out. Healing involves a greater experience of oneness, wholeness, and reconnection with all aspects of your being.[1]

Many of us have known someone who experienced a health problem and, despite the finest medical care (and often a positive initial medical prognosis), got sicker and died. We have also seen people with life-threatening "terminal" diseases who were given up on by their doctors, return from the brink of death to enjoy long, healthy, and productive lives. Most such cases are downplayed by members of the medical profession, because they go against the dominant view that outside agents like drugs, radiation, and surgery are the determining factors in recovering health. The belief that healing occurs primarily from within is incomprehensible.

José's Story

Seven years ago, my friend José was diagnosed with pancreatic cancer, which had spread to the liver. His physician, a prominent oncologist at a major Boston hospital, referred to José as "a sad case" to his colleagues and held out no hope for his recovery. He recommended surgery as the only way to prolong José's life.

José decided to return to his native Brazil, where he was examined by other oncologists at the hospital affiliated with Brazil's finest medical school. They confirmed the original diagnosis and, like the Boston doctor, held out no hope for his recovery. They offered him surgery, radiation, and chemotherapy, which were refused. José, who, as a psychiatrist, had a medical degree, knew that those therapies would kill him. He decided instead to retreat to the countryside, where he embarked on a holistic path to healing that involved intense spiritual and psychological work, using a number of native healing plants. That led to important insights about his life, which brought about major changes in attitude, belief, behavior, and diet, all of which had a positive (and powerful) impact on his health.

José returned to the hospital in Rio for a checkup six months later, where a CAT scan and other tests determined that the cancer had completely disappeared. His doctors were flabbergasted. Since they knew that nearly everyone with advanced pancreatic cancer dies within six months of the initial diagnosis, they simply could not accept evidence of a complete remission, let alone one taking place in the absence of traditional medical therapy. Although they were happy for José (who remains in excellent health after six years), they announced that they must have erred in their original diagnosis and that he didn't have cancer after all! The idea of a complete recovery from pancreatic cancer through holistic healing was inconceivable to them.

Mind–Body Healing

The holistic view of healing teaches that human beings are more than just the physical body and that emotions, thoughts, attitudes, and spirituality play an essential role in healing. Rather than conform to the predominant medical view that there is "one cause" and "one cure" to disease, holism stresses that health and disease depend on a dynamic and often subtle interplay among the physical, emotional, mental, and spiritual aspects of our being, as well as our relationship to the environment in which we live. According to Larry Dossey, M.D., in his book *Space, Time & Medicine:*

> Health is harmony, and harmony has no meaning without the fluid movement of interdependent parts. Like a stream that becomes stagnant when it ceases to flow, harmony and health turn into disease when stasis occurs. We return to the concept of the biodance, the endless streaming of the body-in-flux.[2]

During the past few years, an important new field called *psychoneuroimmunology* has developed. It is concerned with identifying the links between the mind, the brain, and the immune system and determining how they communicate with each other. Researchers have scientifically confirmed that our mind and feelings influence health, while our health has a powerful effect on the mind.

In her book *Good Health in a Toxic World,* Sara Shannon summarizes the major findings of psychoneuroimmunology in understanding the interplay of mind–body healing:

1. Mind-directed, cell-enhancing chemicals communicate directly with the immune system.
2. Mental attitude and mood can alter the course of disease.
3. The mind can "will" changes in the body.
4. Stress-related hormones weaken the immune system.
5. Chemicals made by the immune system communicate with the brain.
6. The brain "talks" to the immune system, and the immune system "talks" to the brain.[3]

These discoveries reveal more than ever before how the way that we view ourselves and life's situations can affect our immune response. For example, let's say that you are about to take a ride on the Cyclone, Coney Island's famous roller coaster. If you take that ride with a sense of dread and terror, your brain will produce a neurochemical called norepinephrine, which can contribute to the risk of high blood pressure, clogging of the arteries, and even heart attack. Fear, hopelessness, and the feeling that "nothing works" have also been linked to the production of neurochemicals by negative thought patterns that can lower immune response and promote the aging process.

However, you can view a ride on the Cyclone in another way. You can become excited at the prospect of the intense speed and look forward to the thrill of "letting go." You can scream with pleasure, and you can marvel at the view of the ocean and the feeling of flight. As a result, your brain produces endorphins and benzodiazepines, two neurochemicals that increase your overall sense of well-being. Other chemicals created by positive feelings toward challenges (known as neurotransmitters) strengthen your immune system, slow down the aging process, and protect you from cancer and a number of viruses.

While these different thoughts and emotions may have a temporary impact on health, chronic, repeated, and habitual thought and emotional patterns can have a far more profound, long-term impact on our well-being. Feelings of fear, hopelessness, worry, and worthlessness all affect our "body–mind" system, however subtle those affects may be. Critical attitudes, beliefs in negative outcomes, anger, resentment, and the belief (whether conscious or not) that "I have no control over my life" have been linked to a number of disease states, including cancer, ulcers, and heart disease. Psychologist Thorwald Dethlefsen and physician Rüdiger Dahlke believe that symptoms are bodily expressions of psychological conflicts.

> Symptoms are many and various, yet they are all expressions of one and the same event which we call "illness," and which always occurs within a person's consciousness. Just as the body cannot live without consciousness, so it cannot become "ill" without consciousness either.[4]

Their excellent book *The Healing Power of Illness* (see resources) examines how understanding the symbolism of certain symptoms can lead us to transform inner conflicts into power agents for healing and growth.

Stress and Distress

Researchers such as Hans Selye, M.D., have found that it is not necessarily the stresses of life that lead to disease, but rather *how we adapt to those stresses.* Much of how we adapt is based on our perspectives on ourselves and our life, many of which are learned from childhood. When a stressful incident appears (whether the loss of a loved one, a difficult task, or a change in economic status), we tend to look at the problem through those old perspectives. If we are stuck in rigid, fixed perspectives about ourselves and the way life "should be," we often find it far more difficult to deal with life's changing events. Instead of adapting to the situation and seeking practical solutions, we may instead feel hopeless, frustrated, and afraid. Rather than being a stimulus for action, a life challenge leads us to fear and paralysis.

In their acclaimed book *Getting Well Again*, Carl Simonton, M.D., Stephanie Matthews-Simonton, and James L. Creighton list a number of common psychological traits of the cancer patients they encountered, which appeared to be precursors to their cancer diagnosis:

- "Experiences in childhood result in decisions to be a certain kind of person." The Simontons believe that as children, we often adopt certain ways of thinking, feeling, and being. Some may be positive and some may be negative, but they result in a certain mind-set that is ingrained upon the personality.

- "The individual is rocked by a cluster of stressful life events." These events, such as a loss of a mate or a job or other position, place critical stress on the individual that threatens personal identity.

- "These stresses create a problem with which the individual does not know how to deal." Very often, the stressful situation goes beyond our established ways of coping, and we feel a loss of control over our situation.

- "The individual sees no way of changing the rules about how he or she must act and so feels trapped and helpless to resolve the problem." We often feel incapable of resolving our problem, which often involves changing the way we view ourselves and the world. This causes us to feel helpless, hopeless, and victimized by outer circumstances.

- "The individual puts distance between himself or herself and the problem, becoming static, unchanging, rigid."[5] When this stage occurs, the individual feels that life no longer has any meaning and, despite outer appearances, feels resigned to his or her fate.

Bio-oxidative Therapies and the Body–Mind

As tools for healing, ozone and hydrogen peroxide can have a powerful effect on our emotional well-being, largely because of their documented analgesic effects. Many people who have used bio-oxidative therapies find that they feel less pain and are not as depressed as they were before. As they place less focus on feeling bad, they experience more energy, optimism, and emotional well-being.

While the psychological benefits of ozone and hydrogen peroxide need to be explored further (research is currently being done by Arthur Janov, Ph.D., the author of the acclaimed book *The Primal Scream*, on how bio-oxidative therapies can be an adjunct to psychological treatment), it is already clear that they can provide a valuable emotional respite from pain and discomfort that one needs to explore new avenues of growth, transformation and healing, in addition to the powerful effects they can have on the physical body.

Disease: A Wake-Up Call to Change

In the context of holistic healing, illness should never be viewed as a punishment or a failure. Instead, disease can be seen as the result of a lack of alignment among the physical, emotional, mental, and spiritual aspects of our being. Rather than being viewed as "bad" or "evil," symptoms are the body's way of telling us that something is wrong. They are a "wake-up call" that tells us that we need to change old attitudes, perspectives, and lifestyle habits that may have contributed to a health problem. To the degree that we are sensitive to our body's subtle messages, we can often deal with a problem before it becomes serious.

Life-threatening diseases such as cancer and AIDS can play a special role in the transformative process. They challenge us to the very core of our being and can mobilize us—like my friend José—to make major changes in personality, thinking, and lifestyle. According to Jason Serinus in *Psychoimmunity and the Healing Process*:

> A diagnosis of AIDS is not necessarily a death sentence; but transforming that diagnosis into an opportunity for healing demands a total commitment. Precisely because the disease is so insidious, it attacks people on the three levels of mind, body and spirit, it must be approached simultaneously on all three levels. The decision to live must be total, involving every thought, every cell, every habit and belief. . . . AIDS represents a real test of who one was and who one chooses to be.[6]

Illness forces us to make choices. While choices based on fear and other limited perspectives often lead to more suffering, those based on knowledge and hope often lead to healing. Those choices may involve greater inner alignment and harmony, changing a destructive emotional or thought pattern, relinquishing resentment, letting go of childhood hurts, and coming to terms with other difficult aspects of one's past.

In their book *Living in Hope*, Cindy Mikluscak-Cooper, R.N., and Emmett E. Miller, M.D., list many of the traits that long-term survivors of AIDS have in common. Many are similar to those of long-term cancer survivors. The ones appearing here are applicable to those suffering from all serious illness, whether life threatening or not. These traits include:

- having a sense of personal responsibility for their health and a sense that they can influence it
- having a sense of purpose in life
- finding new meaning in life as a result of the illness itself
- having previously mastered a life-threatening illness or other life crisis
- having accepted the reality of their diagnosis, yet refusing to believe that it is a death sentence
- having an ability to communicate their concerns to others, including concerns regarding the illness itself
- being assertive and having the ability to say "No"
- having the ability to withdraw from involvements and to nurture themselves
- being sensitive to their body and its needs[7]

Other common traits among long-term AIDS survivors are addressed in Scott J. Gregory's book, *A Holistic Protocol for the Immune System*. Ten points in particular stand out, which are summarized as follows:

1. They had expectations of favorable results regarding their situation.
2. They took charge of their healing and took control of decisions that vitally affected their lives.
3. They developed a sense of humor and learned to laugh.
4. They developed compassion toward others.
5. They were patient in their expectations and did not expect to be healed overnight.

6. They changed their attitudes about themselves and developed a stronger self-image.

7. They realized that there was no one thing that could cure them and sought a combination of life-reinforcing factors and modalities.

8. They had no fear of death—or life.

9. They educated themselves in prevention and treatment.

10. They were fighters.[8]

While healing often leads to a marked improvement in our physical condition, that isn't always the case. Some people, for example, experience healing on psychological or spiritual levels, but physical healing may no longer be possible. They may be too debilitated physically to survive, or they may have the deep realization that their life task is over.

Some years ago, I remember going to the hospital to visit an acquaintance with advanced AIDS who had had a very difficult relationship with his father. An admiral in the navy, the father had never accepted the fact that his son was gay, and they hadn't spoken to each other in years. When he heard of his son's condition, however, the father rushed to his bedside and remained there for two months. During that time, a tremendous amount of healing occurred between father and son, which was often very moving for those of us who visited the hospital on a regular basis. When there appeared to be resolution in their relationship, the son finally decided to "let go" and die.

Self-Nurturing

Although bio-oxidative therapies and adjuncts such as diet and body cleansing assist in the healing process, it is *we* who do the healing. We simply have to allow it to take place. An important component in the process is to create an environment that will facilitate the healing process in our lives. This is not unlike a farmer preparing the soil in expectation of an abundant crop. While this environment varies according to one's personal needs and life situation, it involves three often overlooked aspects of ourselves: our emotional being, our mental being, and our spiritual being. On the following pages, we offer a few ideas that can enhance self-nurturing on emotional, mental, and spiritual levels.

Keep in mind that the subject of this chapter easily deserves an entire book. While the small amount of information provided can help lay the groundwork for healing on all levels, remember that the potentials for healing are limitless, can be adapted to our individual needs, and can be mobilized—in different ways—by everyone.

Nurturing the Emotional Self

Our emotions play an important role in health and disease. While positive feelings produce neurochemicals that strengthen the immune system, negative, repressed, or distorted emotions can decrease immune response and open the door to a variety of health problems. That is why emotional well-being is an important aspect of healing. Rather than try to repress, deny, or control our emotions, we need to nourish and guide them so that they can help us become integrated and whole.

Emotional nurturing can involve creating a support system. This may take the form of being with others who support our healing process, such as relatives or friends. At times, we may need to distance ourselves from those who are not supportive or let them become more aware of our needs and how they might assist us in a positive way. We can also join an organized support group made up of people with health problems similar to our own. Hospitals and social service organizations can often suggest groups that meet locally. The importance of having a support system of that kind cannot be underestimated, especially if one is challenged by a life-threatening disease.

Beauty is also important in emotional healing. Surrounding ourselves with beautiful paintings and prints, or having a vase of fresh flowers in the bedroom or living room, is a wonderful healing gift. Working in the garden, taking a walk in the woods, or sitting by a lake or stream helps stabilize our emotions and gets us more in touch with our natural rhythms. Visit an art museum, watch an inspiring movie, or listen to uplifting music. The possibilities are limited only by our imaginations.

Accepting all of our feelings (including sexual feelings) can be a powerful act of healing. Expressing anger, grief, frustration, or sadness is not always as easy in our culture as the expression of joy, excitement, and affection. But like a river whose current is obstructed, emotions that are blocked tend to become polluted and harmful, since by their very nature, emotions are to be experienced and expressed. Long-term repression of emotions has long been viewed as a factor in a number of common diseases, including cancer, stroke, and heart attack. It probably contributes to less dramatic diseases as well, such as depression and chronic fatigue.

Through meditation, dynamic exercise, and different forms of body-oriented modalities like bioenergetics, Network Chiropractic, and Zero Balancing, we can learn to accept our human emotions and channel them into positive areas of expression.

Many people find that helping others can be a healing emotional gift to everyone involved. Doing volunteer work in a hospital, tutoring a child, or cleaning up a neighborhood park can provide intense satisfaction and the feeling that we are being useful. Those types of activities take us "out of ourselves": We place less emphasis on our own problems and become more involved in our community.

Another important component of emotional nurturing is humor. In his book *Anatomy of an Illness*, Norman Cousins wrote how ten minutes of belly laughter at frequent intervals (he watched Marx Brothers movies and old "Candid Camera" television shows) helped him overcome a life-threatening disease.[9]

Karen Shultz wrote about the healing aspects of hearty, sincere laughter in the anthology *The Essence of Healing.* She says that it allows us to

1. exercise the muscles of the lungs, diaphragm, abdomen, chest and shoulders, stimulating the circulatory system and exercising the breathing muscles;
2. increase the oxygen in our blood;
3. become profoundly self-relaxed—after laughing, the pulse rate, heartbeat and blood pressure drop below normal and the skeletal muscles become deeply relaxed, indicating reduced stress;
4. control pain by increasing production of endorphins, the body's natural pain killers.[10]

Another often overlooked yet very pleasurable form of emotional nourishment is "hug therapy." Dr. David Bresler of the UCLA Pain Control Unit in Los Angeles prescribes a minimum of four hugs a day for men and women to relieve stress and emotional tension.

Perhaps most important, one needs to heal old emotional wounds. Making peace with others, in ways such as forgiving those who have hurt us, asking forgiveness from those we have hurt, letting go of resentment, and especially forgiving ourselves are essential to this process. The books of Louise Hay (see resources) offer valuable tools to those aspects of emotional healing. Twelve-step programs, psychotherapy, body-oriented therapies like bioenergetics and Core Energetics, Pre-Cognitive Re-Education, neurolinguistic programming, yoga, meditation, breathwork, Network Chiropractic, Zero Balancing, and the book *The Twelve Stages of Healing* by Donald Epstein (listed in the resources section) can all facilitate the process of emotional healing.

Nurturing the Mind

At this point in our history, we have access to more information than ever before. While access to information can be valuable, the unrelenting amount of gossip; sensationalism; superficial ideas; and negative, fear-producing concepts from advertising, news reports, and politics creates a type of mental pollution that many of us can do without. It dulls our mental awareness, keeps us living on the periphery, and inhibits our innate healing capacity.

Of particular concern is the constant barrage of negative reports concerning death and disease. Despite Louis Pasteur's advice that "the microbe is nothing; the soil is everything" (meaning that a healthy body will not provide fertile soil for germs to cause disease), news reports and magazine articles often focus on an ever-increasing number of outside agents that will give us cancer, tuberculosis, AIDS, and a myriad of other diseases. This creates a mental environment of fear and hopelessness.

Unless we throw out our radio and television and decide to avoid reading newspapers and magazines, we probably cannot escape this onslaught. Yet we can avoid much of the negative information through our powers of discernment and discrimination. We can choose not to "hook into" initial reports on certain diseases, keeping in mind that many are the result of a limited approach and partial understandings. For example, in the early 1980s we were told that AIDS was an always-fatal disease. After it was found that many patients remained alive and productive five to ten years after diagnosis, the media decided that it wasn't necessarily always fatal after all.

Questioning is an important aspect of mental healing. As children, many of us formed certain ideas about ourselves, our talents, our tasks in life. We also created ideas about other people and the world in which we live. While many of those ideas may have been useful at one time, they may not be useful now. The idea that "my older brother is mean and will beat me up" may have been true when we were five, but at age fifty, it is no longer the case. The idea that "I'm no good at art" may reflect a bad experience in a second-grade art class that still stops us from experiencing our innate creativity. We need to question whether an old concept is still valid or whether it can be changed. As a result, we expand our perspectives, which can bring us new opportunities for understanding and personal growth.

A common negative belief is that because a friend or relative has died of a certain disease, we will also. While we may be genetically predisposed to certain health problems, that does not mean that they will manifest as symptoms. A friend once put it to me this way: "Just because my father had cancer doesn't mean that I will. I don't think like him, eat like him, or live like him. We are different people." In addition, we need to be aware that the body we have now is not the same one we had five or ten years ago, since every cell of the body is in the process of dying while others are being regenerated. The health of future cells, and therefore the future health of our entire body–mind, is dependent on how we live, eat, and think in the present.

The Great Epidemic

Negative thinking has become epidemic in our world. During the course of every day, each of us may be the source of hundreds of negative thoughts concerning impending disasters (large and small), as well as worries about negative outcomes; images of being undeserving or un-worthy of good things in life; ideas of being rejected, offended, or betrayed; and exaggerated notions of the importance of everyday aches and pains.

Thought is a powerful force, and thinking helps create the world in which we live. Given that billions of people probably produce hundreds of negative thoughts each day, it should be no wonder that we live in a world that is violent, polluted, unhappy, and in great need of healing.

Negative thinking is a totally useless activity. It is anchored in the past and projected into the future, avoiding the truth of the present moment, which is the only reality. By becoming aware of when we create negative thoughts, we can begin to stop contributing to the store-house of negative thinking in the world.

There are many good books and courses available on positive think-ing. Yet simply by becoming more aware of our negative thinking and understanding how harmful it is for ourselves and others, we gradually discover that our thought patterns can change. Even a simple affirmation like "Today, I will only have positive thoughts" every time we catch ourselves in negative thinking can help transform a negative pattern into one that supports the healing process, if only for a moment.

Books that educate us and empower us in our healing journey are powerful sources of mental nurturing. Many of the books included in the resources section provide that type of support and show how we can recover and maintain our health. In addition, inspirational readings from holy books, "twelve-step" meditation books, and stories about the healing journeys of others can inspire us and help create positive thoughts. Understanding the hidden meanings of fairy tales, studying books of ancient wisdom, and learning about the holistic healing practices of both traditional and modern cultures are also ways to enhance mental nurturing. Remember, however, that nurturing of the mind should not be done at the expense of the emotions. Both need to be nurtured to achieve harmonious fulfillment in our lives.

Creative Visualization

Creative visualization is often used in healing. There are a number of excellent books dealing with visualization, available in many bookstores and libraries. Louise Hay outlines the three basic parts of a positive visualization, which can be adapted to individual needs:

1. An image of the problem or pain or dis-ease, or the dis-eased part of the body.
2. An image of a positive force eliminating this problem.
3. An image of the body being rebuilt to perfect health, then seeing the body move through life with ease and energy.[11]

Positive visualization can incorporate literal images, symbolic images related to treatment, and abstract images. One universal image is a bright, white, healing light, which one can imagine shining around (and through) every aspect of one's being. A powerful tool to aid this type of creative visualization is "The Divine Light Invocation Mantra" taught by Swami Sivananda Radha:

I am created by Divine Light
I am sustained by Divine Light

> I am protected by Divine Light
>
> I am surrounded by Divine Light
>
> I am ever growing into Divine Light.[12]

Some people may wish to visualize being healed by Jesus Christ or the Healing Buddha, while others may wish to incorporate saints, yogis, angels, or other spiritual beings into their healing visualizations.

Finally, mental healing involves becoming aware of what is really important to us. Possessions, prestige, money in the bank, and a country-club membership may be nice to have, but many people facing serious illness soon realize that they are not as important as they once thought. Good relationships, inner peace, connection with a Higher (or Deeper) Power, and a sense of purpose in life often move to the foreground during a healing crisis.

One of the benefits of illness is that it brings us into reality. We begin to discern the true from the false, and the essence from the superficial. We begin to see the kind of life we truly want to have and often come upon the ways needed to achieve it.

Spiritual Nurturing

Spirituality is viewed to have little impact on healing by most physicians, yet it can provide the foundation for deep healing to take place. People know the source of spirituality by many names: God, Allah, the Inner Light, Organizing Wisdom, the Divine Teacher. Whatever label we choose to give that Source, spirituality involves tapping into the deeper levels of our being where inner wisdom and love can be found. As we connect to that love–wisdom, we are able to create a greater sense of harmony and alignment among all aspects of our being. That allows the healing process to occur.

If we participate in self-nurturing on the emotional and mental levels, spiritual nurturing is a natural result, because all are interconnected and interrelated. However, there are many specific ways to enhance healing through spiritual means that can be both inspiring and empowering.

Many of us engage in spiritual nurturing on special occasions, such as when we go to our house of worship, or when we are experiencing a crisis. While that is important, many teachers have stressed the importance of becoming aware of the sacred in everyday life. This involves not only understanding the spiritual component in daily challenges and viewing our immediate situation in the context of a greater or deeper reality, but also learning how to see the sacred in the world around us, including in other people, animals, and nature.

Trees and flowers are an often overlooked source of spiritual nourishment in our modern, industrialized world. Yet many of our ancestors—like members of indigenous and traditional cultures today—have long appreciated the healing power of trees and used them for healing all levels of their being. In addition to their beauty, trees are strong, graceful, adaptable, and deeply grounded in what Native Americans call "the Earth Mother." By developing a close relationship with trees (many of us, in fact, had a "favorite tree" as a child), we can share their natural qualities.

There are many ways to commune with trees: resting in their shade, standing or leaning against their trunks, and even hugging them can open us to a source of Earth energy we rarely experience. In my book *Sacred Trees* (Sierra Club Books, 1994), I've included more detailed information about the spiritual and healing aspects of trees and how we can partake of them.

Another powerful, yet often overlooked, natural source of spiritual nourishment is flowers. Although most of us like flowers, we do not take the time to appreciate them. Flowers offer strength, grace, color, pattern, and dazzling beauty. Flowers have a lot to teach us about life. A wildflower growing (and thriving) in a crack in the sidewalk shows us how one can survive and thrive under even the most difficult circumstances. A new flower can reveal the beauty involved in openness and vulnerability. A flower in full bloom can tell us the value of giving fully of ourselves without holding back or being concerned with what others may say. A dying flower can reveal the grace and understanding of accepting death as a natural part of our life cycle.

Finally, prayer can be a powerful force in healing. It is an expression of yearning from deep within our being to realize our connection with the Source of all life. Prayer acknowledges our union with that Source, which is both outside of us and deep within. Prayer has been likened to our sending off radiowaves of goodness into the world and beyond.

Prayers may take many forms. They may involve repeating a sacred word or phrase, they may be prayers for the healing of self or of a loved one, or they may articulate a special blessing to the world. The following Buddhist prayer is especially beautiful:

May all people and all forms of life be surrounded with Infinite Love and Compassion. Particularly do we send forth loving thoughts to those in suffering and sorrow, to all those in doubt and ignorance, to all who are striving to attain the truth, and to those whose feet are standing close to the great change we call death, we send forth oceans of Love, Wisdom and Compassion.

Whenever we pray, we open ourselves to the possibility of deep healing blessing. It is a humble act that is grounded in our desire to realize our oneness and wholeness. That is, in effect, the essential goal of healing.

13

OXYGEN PRODUCTS, SERVICES, AND APPLICATIONS

This chapter explores some of the growing variety of oxygen-therapy-related products, services, and applications that have become available to the general public. Our intent is not to promote or endorse any particular product and applications, but to explore their uses and value to the consumer.

Ozone Generators

We mentioned before that ozone is produced by humans by passing an electrical charge through a specially built condenser containing oxygen. A number of different types of ozone generators are available commercially.

Ultraviolet (UV) ozone generators are less expensive than other types, but their output of ozone is low. However, the need to change the UV bulb (approximately every ten thousand hours) can drive up the cost of the equipment over time. Ozone output is not constant due to deterioration of the UV bulb. Ozone production can be regulated only by air flow.

When nitrogen in the air (air is made up of approximately 80 percent nitrogen) is exposed to a high-voltage discharge (including that made with most ozone generators), it will react with oxygen and form small amounts of NOx, or nitrogen oxides, a group of nitrogen and oxygen chemical compounds, including nitrous oxide (N_2O) and nitric oxide (NO). From this group of chemical compounds, we also find the highly toxic nitrogen dioxide NO_2, which is derived by oxidation of nitric oxide. This gas is highly toxic to the lungs and is used in the production of nitric acid.

However, when ozone is created from pure oxygen and discharged into the air, it does not react with nitrogen. Ultraviolet systems with a wavelength 194 nm and shorter will produce ozone, but no NOx even if air (as opposed to pure oxygen) is used as the feed gas.

Cold plasma machines represent the middle range in both cost and ozone output. They do not require replacement of the ozone-producing cell, and their ozone output can be retained at a constant level. Ozone production is possible to regulate only by air flow. However, when air is used as a feed gas, it can produce NOx.

Corona discharge generators cost more than the other systems and provide the highest output of ozone. Output is constant, and one does not need to periodically replace the cell. One can regulate ozone production by air flow and/or by changing the high-voltage discharge (voltage or frequency). Like the cold plasma machine, it will produce NOx when air is used as feed gas.

This type of generator is also referred to as a *hot spark*-type ozone generator. However, with the availability of high-quality dielectric materials and semiconductors, properly designed corona discharge-type ozone generators produce far less heat than their ancestors. Over the past few years, they have become popular for their wide variety of applications due to their high ozone output and ability to regulate ozone output independently from air flow.

Air Purifiers

Many people have also become interested in commercial air purifiers that generate ozone. The manufacturers often claim that these ozone generators provide additional oxygen for breathing, while killing bacteria, fungi, molds, yeasts, and dust mites. They are also supposed to remove harmful contaminants from the air, such as cigarette smoke and other airborne toxins.

The use of these machines is controversial. Many scientists believe that inhaling ozone in any amount is harmful to one's health, although there is some question regarding what constitutes a harmful concentration. As mentioned earlier, Russian physicians have introduced therapeutic ozone into the lungs of critically ill patients without adverse reactions. Many lay advocates of bio-oxidative therapies believe that using ozone generators to purify the air is both safe and effective. One such machine was used to purify the air in the exhibition area at a conference on bio-oxidative therapies I attended several years ago. Ed McCabe, the author of O_2xygen Therapies and the foremost exponent of the health benefits of therapeutic hydrogen peroxide and ozone, has been using a portable ozone generator to purify air for years, both at home and during his lecture tours. He finds it particularly beneficial in cleaning the air of stuffy hotel rooms.

There are a number of points to consider when using an air purifier that generates ozone. Den Rasplicka, an engineer and the founder of Ozone Services (see resources), points out that electronic equipment, such as computers, television sets, compact disk players, and VCRs, is sensitive to ozone. Ozone can enter air vents or cooling ducts and may damage delicate components. In addition, some components contain a printed circuit board that lacks a solder mask, which is a protective layer over the traces on the board. These traces can suffer from oxidation caused by ozone. Ozone can also oxidize drive belts in VCRs, cassette players, and compact disc players, because these belts are made with rubber or latex, which oxidize easily.

He also advises that there are two ways to deal with household odors with ozone. One can treat the air alone with very low levels of ozone or the source of the odor through heavy, prolonged periods of ozonation. When the second option is chosen, the area to be ozonated should be carefully prepared before treatment: Sensitive electronic components like television sets, VCRs, compact disc players, and computers—as well as paintings and plants—should be removed before treating the room.

Some people are very sensitive to even small amounts of nitrogen dioxide (NO_2). In general, healthy people will not have any problems with an air purifier in the room. However, Mr. Rasplicka notes that people who are sick (or those with severely depressed immune systems) are sensitive to it. The two major symptoms that show that one is sensitive to NO_2 are sudden, severe headache or dizziness. Individuals who are sensitive to even extremely low concentrations of nitrogen dioxide will not be able to be present when the air purification unit is running. For these people, rooms treated by ozone air purifiers will have to be unoccupied and properly ventilated after treatment. The ambient air is not really purified with ozone, the benefit comes primarily from the purification of walls, ceilings, carpeting, bedding, and upholstery, which serve as a breeding ground for air-borne bacteria, noxious gases, dust mite feces, mildew, mold, and other allergens and irritants.[1]

Although properly designed air purifiers will emit safe amounts of ozone, it is important to be aware of ozone levels in the ambient air in parts per million (ppm). A concentration of 0.001 to 0.12 ppm are typically found in the natural atmosphere. These levels of concentration vary with altitude, atmospheric conditions, and locale. The Environmental Protection Agency set the level of the national primary and secondary air quality standards also at 0.12 ppm.[2] A limit of 0.040 ppm is said to be the maximum set by the Canadian Standard Association for devices designed for household use, while 0.050 ppm is the maximum allowable ozone concentration recommended by the American Society of Heating, Refrigerating, and Air Conditioning Engineers in an air-conditioned and ventilated space. It is also the maximum ozone concentration produced by electronic air cleaners and similar residential devices according to the proposed amendment of the Federal Food, Drug, and Cosmetic Act. Ozone levels higher than this should be considered unsafe. Ozone levels can be monitored. A new generation of ozone air purifiers that have a built-in ozone level sensor to help determine the amount of ozone in the air are produced. However, an alternative low-cost option to monitor or assess ambient ozone levels present are ozone test strips, which are used the same way as standard pH test strips. More sophisticated ozone testers, monitors, and controllers are also available, but are often expensive.

Although more research needs to be done in studying ozone generation and air purification, a growing number of hospitals, hotels, restaurants, and offices are moving toward ozone, even to the extent of installing large permanent ozone generation systems in their buildings. A 1996 article in the *New Hampshire Business Review* described the benefits of purifying air with ozone:

> Ozone is a fast-acting cleaning and oxidizing agent. Ozone eliminates office odors by chemically neutralizing them, not covering them up with another, albeit more pleasant, smell. Ozone helps rid the air of many common causes of inhaled allergies, and it kills mold, mildew, spores and pollen. Ozone also kills bacteria and many viruses and airborne diseases. This makes your office a healthier and more pleasant workplace and helps eliminate sick building syndrome.[3]

Ozonated Drinking Water

We mentioned earlier that ozonization is an important method of purifying water and is used by thousands of municipalities around the world to remove impurities and pathogens from drinking water. A growing number of individuals have decided to ozonate their own drinking water for both disinfection and therapeutic reasons. While drinking ozonated water is a good idea, such applications require specific concentrations of ozone. In addition, ozonated water has a definite shelf life, after which it will lose its therapeutic value.

Scientists view ozone application in water in terms of "oxygen reduction potential" or ORP, which is measured in millivolts (mV) of DC. The following list offers a general idea of levels of ORP needed for different ozone applications:

200–400 ORP: cooling towers and aquaculture

400–600 ORP: hot tubs, swimming pools, general water-treatment applications

600–800 ORP: water disinfection

800 ORP and up: water sterilization

900 ORP and up: water with residual ozone levels able to deliver a therapeutic effect.[4]

Ozone tends to decompose in water over time. The shelf life of ozonated water depends not only on elapsed time after ozonation, but on the type of container it is stored in. The following chart shows the shelf life of ozonated water in three types of containers: a 1500-ml glass chamber that is 2.5 inches in diameter and 23 feet high, a 1000-ml glass container 4 inches in diameter and 6 inches high, and a 1000-ml plastic container. These figures were determined through laboratory analysis by Zdenek Rasplicka of Ozone Services and were kindly provided by him.

Ozonated Water for Swimming Pools and Hot Tubs

Many companies install ozone equipment for swimming pools and hot tubs. As opposed to using large amounts of chlorine, which has been

Figure 13.1. Ozonated water shelf life. (Reprinted courtesy of Ozone Services.)

linked to cancer and is harmful to the environment, ozone is readily absorbed in water, can have therapeutic value to those who use the pool or spa, and is environmentally friendly. In addition, ozone is more efficient at killing bacteria, fungi, parasites, toxic chemicals, and other waterborne contaminants: While chlorine slowly seeps into the cell wall of the contaminants, ozone ruptures the cell wall and shatters the molecular bonds of the complex chains of the contaminants, destroying them quickly and completely. In addition, the less spa or pool equipment exposure to chemicals, the less maintenance, and the need for bromine floaters, chlorine, water clarifiers, and other chemicals are virtually eliminated. There are few disadvantages to using ozone purification systems; however, some have reported that water bugs and frogs, who rarely appear in chlorinated water, are attracted to pools and hot tubs cleaned by ozone. While this is a minor nuisance, it makes one realize that chlorine and other chemicals in the water do not create an environment amenable to living beings. Ozone in standard dosages for swimming pools (400–475 ORP) does not kill algae, while a dose higher than 500 ORP will.

Not all pool or hot tub filtering systems are designed to work with ozone gas purification; a knowledgeable spa contractor can determine how your system can be reconfigured, if necessary. As with any water purification system, make sure that you purchase an ozone generator for pool or spa use from a reputable dealer who has extensive experience with ozone purification systems.

What about hydrogen peroxide in pools and hot tubs? While utilizing 35 percent hydrogen peroxide in a swimming pool on a regular basis can be expensive, adding food-grade hydrogen peroxide to the water in a hot tub is both safe and practical. Den Rasplicka recommends that concentrations of 35 percent hydrogen peroxide should be 50–80 ppm concentration. Food-grade hydrogen peroxide is available in gallon (and larger) containers from dozens of sources, including vendors of agricultural supplies. Test strips to measure hydrogen peroxide concentrations are available commercially as well.

The Oxygen Bar

Another recent development has been the appearance of the "oxygen bar." The first one in North America (the O_2 Spa Bar) opened in Toronto in 1996,[5] and others are sprouting up in trendy neighborhoods in many other cities, including Vancouver, New York, Los Angeles, and Detroit. Modeled in part after the "air stations" located in polluted downtown areas of Tokyo and Beijing, where oxygen is dispensed to beleaguered clients through a vending machine, the oxygen bars offer a relaxing environment with comfortable seating, soft music, and healthy refreshments.

In addition to offering respite from the physical and psychological stresses of city life, these spas offer clients supplemental oxygen (in the form of 99.9 percent pure medical–grade oxygen) administered through the nostrils for about twenty to thirty minutes. While receiving their spa treatment, clients may listen to music, read, or watch a video over a cup of herbal tea. Proponents of supplemental oxygen point out that it is used therapeutically to treat over a dozen health complaints, including migraines and cluster headaches. They also mention that supplemental oxygen can be beneficial to healthy people as well.

As can be expected, skeptics abound. They point out that there is no clinical evidence that supplemental oxygen is of value to healthy people and that overuse can be hazardous to health. Some even feel that administering supplemental oxygen is a medical procedure and should be regulated as such. However, the owners of oxygen bars generally make no therapeutic claims for oxygen to avoid being accused of practicing medicine without a license. The basic pitch is one of comfort and renewal. According to a publicity notice for a new oxygen bar in New York City:

> Now imagine yourself sitting on a soft leather reclining chair in a beautiful cozy room with a couple of friends, listening to relaxing music, breathing pure, cool oxygen from a small, comfortable plastic tube under your nose. After a short time, when finished, most will walk out feeling relaxed, rested, awake and refreshed, ready to go out to the gym or to party. They've improved their health and leave feeling great.[6]

Oxygenated Bottled Waters

With approximately seven times more oxygen than found in ordinary water, commercial oxygenated water producers claim that their beverage provides increased endurance, improved athletic performance, and an overall energy boost. Using patented technology, extra oxygen (approximately 70 mg/liter) is added to ordinary purified water. The reputed energy boost is due to the increased amount of oxygen in the blood.

As with oxygen spas, skeptics find claims about oxygenated water hard to swallow. They question how the intestine is able to absorb extra oxygen by drinking oxygen-enriched water, while proponents of oxygenated water claim that the patented process facilitates oxygen absorption through the colon. I have tried oxygenated water (marketed under the label "O_2 Water") and found it both thirst quenching and better tasting than other types of bottled water. Despite the manufacturer's claims that athletes have improved their performance after drinking this water, I did not experience the promised extra boost of energy after drinking it.

Oxygenation Products

A growing number of bio-oxidative and oxygenation products, including oxygen-saturated skin creams, stabilized oxygen dietary supplements, skin sprays, and colon cleansers are becoming increasingly available to the general public through mail-order companies and health-food stores. Some of the most popular are marketed as food supplements and go by trademarked names like Cellfood, Liquid Life, Oxygen for Life, Chelo Zone, Oxy-Gen, Colo Zone, OxyBliss, OxyCleanse, Bioxy Cleanse, Oxy Aloe, SuperOxy, Homozone, and OxyToddy. Some of the products claim to contain small amounts of hydrogen peroxide, but are far more palatable to ingest than drops of food-grade hydrogen peroxide in a glass of water. Many users have reported that these products provide added energy and have helped them maintain good health; some even claim that these products have helped them overcome disease when traditional allopathic medications had failed them.

Even within the oxygen therapy community, these products have their critics. They point out that many commercial bio-oxidative and oxygenation products are expensive and are sold through high-pressure "multi-level marketing" techniques where a person sells the product to a customer and then contracts the customer to sell the product to others at a commission. In addition to commissions on direct sales, the original seller (now a distributor) earns a commission on sales made by the customers he or she recruits. While such marketing methods are not illegal, the quest for high commissions can lead to high-pressure sales tactics and exaggerated health claims.

With the possible exceptions of ozonated olive oil, 35 percent food-grade hydrogen peroxide (diluted in water and taken internally or added to bathwater), Heritage's Oxy Aloe, and Dr. Donsbach's SuperOxy and Oxy-Gen products (which are made with magnesium peroxide), most products focus on increasing *oxygenation* as opposed to *oxidation*. Some skeptics point out that a session of deep yogic breathing or a twenty-minute aerobic workout would oxygenate the body more efficiently (and at lower cost) than the use of commercial oxygenation products.

Another criticism regarding these products is that they have not undergone rigorous laboratory and clinical trials to verify their safety and effectiveness. This is a valid concern, which also applies to the plethora of vitamins, mineral supplements, and herbal preparations that have flooded the health-care marketplace. This does not mean that oxidative and oxygenation products are neither safe nor effective; in-deed, some of them have been available for many years and many people swear by them. However, until objective laboratory and clinical evidence is made available to the consumer, perhaps the best yardstick is careful examination of health claims with one's common sense. In addition, consider using a product through recommendation of people you trust who have already tried it and who hopefully do not have a financial stake in the product.

Hydrogen Peroxide in the Kitchen and Garden

We mentioned earlier that 35 percent hydrogen peroxide diluted in water can be used for bathing and as a skin spray. However, many have discovered that it can be helpful in both the kitchen and the garden. The following practical suggestions have been gleaned from a variety of sources:

To make ³/₄ pint of 3 percent hydrogen peroxide solution using 35 percent food-grade hydrogen peroxide, mix 1 ounce of 35 percent hydrogen peroxide into 11 ounces of distilled water. If you spill food-grade hydrogen peroxide on your skin, rinse immediately with warm water and avoid contact with eyes. When you store hydrogen peroxide in the refrigerator, clearly mark the container so you do not mistake it for water.

To clean vegetables and fruit, add ¼ cup of your 3 percent hydrogen peroxide mixture to a sink filled with cold water. Wash the vegetables thoroughly, rinse, and drain. Either consume the vegetables immediately or pat dry and store in the refrigerator. Another method involves spraying the fruits and vegetables with the 3 percent mixture of hydrogen peroxide. Rinse with cold water and drain. This process is said to prolong freshness.

For washing dishes in an automatic dishwasher, add 2 ounces of 3 percent hydrogen peroxide to your regular washing formula. You can also keep a spray bottle of your hydrogen peroxide solution in the kitchen to be sprayed on countertops and appliances. It will disinfect surfaces and will also give the kitchen a clean, fresh smell. This process can also be used to freshen the refrigerator and children's lunchboxes.

Some farmers are reported to have used hydrogen peroxide on their crops. To foliar feed crops, add 16 ounces of 35 percent hydrogen peroxide to 20 gallons of water. Spray on plants early in the morning, while the plant pores are open. This should be enough to spray one acre of crops.

To facilitate seed germination, add 1 ounce of 3 percent hydrogen peroxide into a pint of distilled water. Soak the seeds for 8 hours. This method is reputed to increase the rate of seed germination by 30 percent.

To make plant insecticide, mix 8 ounces or more of 3 percent hydrogen peroxide to 1 gallon of water with 8 ounces of molasses or white sugar. It has been found that blackstrap molasses works better than sugar; it seems to allow the mixture to better adhere to the plant.

To increase the growth of plants, add 1 ounce of 3 percent hydrogen peroxide to a quart of water (or add 16 drops of 35 percent hydrogen peroxide to 1 quart of water). Water or mist plants with this solution. Good results can even be seen by adding just a tablespoonful of 3 percent hydrogen peroxide to 1 gallon of water. Farmers are also watering the ground around fruit trees, adding 6 to 8 ounces of 3 percent H_2O_2 to a gallon of water, which can also be used as a spray. To increase the longevity of cut flowers, add a few drops of 3 percent hydrogen peroxide per cup of water.

Tropical fish enthusiasts have found that adding a maximum of 1 ounce of 35 percent food-grade hydrogen peroxide to 20 gallons of water will help disinfect the aquarium water and reduce fungal growth on fish.

RESOURCES

Networking

OxyTherapy on Internet
Internet e-mail access: amadis@oxytherapy.com
Website: http://www.oxytherapy.com

Subscribe to a free on-line mailing list about bio-oxidative therapies for the prevention and treatment of immune diseases. OxyTherapy has hundreds of members worldwide who can communicate directly with each other about their questions and experiences with oxygen therapies. OxyTherapy.com maintains an electronic forum that provides information about all forms of oxygen/ozone therapies; a database of people, products and events; and an on-line library of files available through FTP (File Transfer Protocol). To subscribe to the mailing list, send a request to majordomo@oxytherapy.com. In the body of your message, include the word "SUBSCRIBE LIST."

North American Organizations

International Oxidative Medicine Association (IOMA)
P.O. Box 891954
Oklahoma City, OK 73109
Tel: (405) 634-7855
Fax: (405) 634-7320

Sponsors yearly international conference and maintains a list of medical practitioners utilizing bio-oxidative therapies around the world. IOMA also conducts training seminars for physicians, funds research in bio-oxidative therapies, and distributes information about these therapies worldwide. It was formerly known as the International Bio-Oxidative Medicine Foundation (IBOMF)

International Association for Oxygen Therapy
P.O. Box 1360
Priest River, ID 83856
Tel: (208) 448-2504
Fax: (208) 448-2657

Formerly the Eastern Association for Oxygen Therapy, this organization was originally founded by the Institut Für Sauerstoff Heilvahfahren in Germany. A source of information about oxygen therapies, especially products developed by Dr. F. M. Blass like Homozone, a product that promotes colon cleansing.

The International Ozone Association, Inc.
Pan American Group
31 Strawberry Hill Avenue
Stamford, CT 06902
Tel: (203) 348-3542
Fax: (203) 967-4845
Website: www.int-ozone-assoc.org/

A network for information and technology transfer in all areas relating to ozone (including medical ozone). Publishes quarterly journal and other literature. Sponsors a variety of conferences around the world.

Keep Hope Alive
P.O. Box 27041
West Allis, WI 53227
Website: www.execpc.com/~keephope/keephope.html

An organization offering strategies related to diet, ozone, and other natural therapies for those infected with HIV and other immune-related problems. Publishes *Positive Health News* and the acclaimed book *AIDS Control Diet* by Mark Konlee, now under the title *How to Reverse Immune Dysfunction*. Has also assembled a collection of articles about medical ozone taken from medical journals, available for purchase. For monthly recorded message updates, call (414) 548-4344.

Physicians Committee for Responsible Medicine
5100 Wisconsin Avenue, N.W., Suite 404
Washington, DC 20016
Website: www.pcrm.org

While not involved with bio-oxidative therapies, this group introduced the New Four Food Groups and promotes preventive health strategies, higher standards for ethics and effectiveness in research, and alternatives to animal research. Publishes *Good Medicine.*

Ann Wigmore Foundation
Ann Wigmore Institute
196 Commonwealth Avenue
Boston, MA 02116

Ann Wigmore was the chief proponent of a natural lifestyle using raw foods and living foods (such as sprouts and wheat grass) to maintain and recover good health. She worked with many patients with cancer, heart disease, and AIDS, often with impressive results. A number of bio-oxidative practitioners have recommended her program for people undergoing therapy with ozone and hydrogen peroxide. Both the foundation (in Boston) and the institute (in Puerto Rico) offer commuter and resident programs teaching people how to use living foods.

European Organizations

The International Ozone Association
International Coordinating Office
83 Avenue Foch
75116 Paris, France

This is the head office of the association that coordinates their international programs around the world.

Gesellschaft fur Ozon- und Sauerstoff-Anwendungen (G.O.S.)
Klagenfurterstrasse 4
Feuerbach
70469 Stuttgart, Germany

Provides a list of ozone practitioners in Europe.

Publications

Townsend Letter for Doctors and Patients
911 Tyler Street
Port Townsend, WA 98368
Website: www. tldp.com/index.html

A magazine written primarily by and for health-care professionals, *The Townsend Letter* explores alternative and complementary therapies for the prevention and cure of disease. Packed with information about herbs, nutrition, homeopathy, and other modalities, every issue has one or two articles about bio-oxidative therapies.

Positive Health News
HIV Treatment News
Keep Hope Alive
P.O. Box 27041
West Allis, WI 53227

These excellent newletters are edited by Mark Konlee, the author of *How to Reverse Immune Dysfunction.* Published several times a year, they focus primarily on the use of bio-oxidative therapies for the prevention and treatment of HIV-related problems, although other natural approaches are discussed as well.

Manufacturers and Distributors of Ozone Generators and Other Oxygen Therapy Products

North America

Ozone Services
390 Silver Queen Road
Burton, B.C. VOG IEO Canada
Tel: (250) 265-4461
Fax: (250) 265-4482
E-mail: ozoneden@o3zone.com
Website: www.o3zone.com/ozoneser

Manufactures and distributes ozone generators, steam cabinets, shower equipment, ozonated oil, and supplies for water purification and medical use. Sponsors Silver Creek Ozone Centre, providing ozone training, educational seminars, and lectures on altternative therapies. Also sponsors *Ozone Gateway* (http://www.o3zone.com/index.html), an on-line directory of ozone-related information, products, and services; including a specialized "Ozone in Cuba" section (http://www.o3zone.com/Cuba) with news of the latest developments and advancements at the Ozone Research Center in Havana.

PlasmaFire
7186-205 Street
Langley, B.C. V2Y 1T1 Canada
Tel: (604) 532-9596
Website: www.plasmafire.com

Manufactures and distributes ozone generators, steam cabinets, and supplies for water purification and medical use.

Family Health News
9845 N.E. Second Avenue
Miami Shores, FL 33138
Tel: (800) 284-6263; (305) 759-8710
Website: www.familyhealthnews.com

Distributes a broad range of oxygen related products, including nutritional supplements, books and tapes, ozone generators, ozonated olive oil, stabilized oxygen products, and hydrogen peroxide. Request a sample copy of their informative magazine and catalog.

FutureMed Incorporated
P.O. Box 13837
Scottsdale, AZ 85260
Tel: (800) 800-8849

Distributes a wide range of health-related products, including stabilized oxygen, books, oxygen enhancement, food supplements, and ozone generators for air purification. Request a catalog.

Crossroads Internet Store
Tel: (800) 635-5823
Website:www.oxytherapy.com/sponsors/crossroads/home.html

Sells a wide variety of oxygen products through the Internet, including books, tapes, oxygen enhancement supplements, air and water purification systems, ozone generators, and accessories.

BioQuest Imports
P.O. Box 27104, 1395 Marine Drive
West Vancouver, B.C. V7T 2XB, Canada
Tel: (604) 925-4728
Fax: (604) 922-4649

Distributors of ozone generators, food supplements, and stabilized oxygen products, including Bioxy Cleanse.

Pegasus
P.O. Box 1066
Evart, MI 49631
Tel: (616) 832-1879

Distributes ozone generators and steam cabinets.

Actual Water Services
1415 Crown Street
Vancouver, B.C. V7J 1G4, Canada
Tel: (604) 986-3306

Manufactures and distributes specialized equipment for colon therapy and ozone applications.

Care Tech Industries, Inc.
St. Petersburg, FL
Tel: (800) 700-3327, (813) 393-3327
Website: www.odatus.com

Manufactures and distributes Odatus brand air purifiers, for home or office use and for commercial buildings, as well as air quality sampling kits.

Summertime Products (regional distributor)
4700 South 900 E., Suite 30–112
Salt Lake City, UT 84117
Tel: (800) 578-7035, (801) 266-0595

Distributes O_3zonator brand air purifiers.

Oxyfresh Worldwide, Inc.
P.O. Box 3723
Spokane, WA 99220
Tel: (509) 924-4999

Manufactures and distributes Oxyfresh Air brand air purifiers.

Alpine Industries
511 Second Avenue, P.O. Box 175
Goodhue, MN 55027
Tel: (800) 369-1297

Manufactures and distributes Alpine Living Air brand air purifiers.

Europe

Dr. J. Hansler GmbH
Nordring 8
76473 Iffezheim, Germany
Tel: (49) 7229 30460

Manufactures and distributes Ozonosan ozone genetors for water purification and medical applications.

Kastner Praxisbedarf GmbH
Berliner Ring 40
7550 Rastatt, Germany
Tel: (49) 7222 33053

Manufactures and distributes Ozomed ozone generators for water purification and medical applications.

Multiossigen srl
Viale Zavaritt 152
24020 Gorle (Bg), Italy
Tel: (39) 35 299573, 035 300903 (within Italy)

Manufactures and distributes medical ozone equipment and supplies.

Medozons
150 Gorky Street
603000 Nizhni Novgorod, Russia
Tel: (7) 8312 358200
E-mail: pov@infotel.nnov.su

Manufactures and distributes medical ozone generators and supplies.

Wilhelm Schmidding GmbH & Co.
Emdener Strasse 10
50735 Cologne, Germany
Tel: (49) 221 717401

Manufactures industrial ozone equipment.

Ozonia International
65. avenue du Mont Valerien
92500 Rueil-Malmaison, France
Tel: (33) 1 47 10 06 00
Tel: (804) 756-0500 (US), (44) 1895 82 03 03 (U.K.)
Manufactures industrial ozone equipment.

Videos

Ozone and the Politics of Medicine
Threshold Film, Inc.
#301-356 East Sixth Avenue
Vancouver, B.C. V5T 1K1, Canada
Tel: (604) 873-4626
    (800) 216-4403

A professionally produced and provocative documentary on how the U.S. government views ozone in the treatment of AIDS and other diseases. Available from Threshold Film or *The Family Health News* (address on page 224).

Oxygen Therapies Introductory Video
A two-hour video of Ed McCabe's first Australian lecture tour. Available from *Crossroads* and *The Family Health News* (address on page 226).

Books

On Bio-oxidative Therapies

Donsbach, Kurt W., *Wholistic Cancer Therapy* and *Oxygen–Peroxides–Ozone* (Tulsa: Rockland Corporation, 1992 and 1993). Short booklets about Dr. Donsbach's work with these natural therapies. Available at many natural-food stores.

Douglass, William Campbell, *Hydrogen Peroxide, Medical Miracle* (Atlanta: Second Opinion Publishing, 1994). A small book describing the original work with hydrogen peroxide of Drs. Farr, Douglass, and others. Many patient testimonials and case histories. Available at bookstores and from *The Family Health News* (address on page 224).

McCabe, Ed, *O$_2$xygen Therapies* (Morrisville, N.Y.: Energy Publications,

1988). A comprehensive book about hydrogen peroxide, ozone, and related products. Available at bookstores and from *The Family Health News* (address on page 224).

Rilling, Siegfried, and Renate Viebahn, *The Use of Ozone in Medicine* (Heidelberg: Haug Publishers, 1987). An excellent guide for practitioners. A new edition, with slight revisions, was published by Haug under Dr. Viebahn's name in 1994. Available from Medicina Biologica, 2937 Flanders St., Portland, OR 97232.

On Natural and Complementary Therapies (Including Diet)

Gawler, Ian, *You Can Conquer Cancer* (Wellingborough: Thorsons Publishing, 1987). A self-help guide to recovering from cancer by someone who's "been there." Includes information on diet and other healing strategies.

Gray, Robert, *The Colon Health Handbook* (Oakland: Rockridge Publishing Company, 1982). A booklet about colon cleansing and intestinal health. Widely available.

Gregory, Scott J., *A Holistic Protocol for the Immune System* (Joshua Tree, Calif.: Tree of Life Publications, 1992). A comprehensive manual for patients with HIV/ARC (AIDS Related Complex)/AIDS, including advice on how to deal with opportunistic infections through natural means.

Konlee, Mark, *How to Reverse Immune Dysfunction* (W. Allis, Wisc: Keep Hope Alive, 1997). An excellent resource about nutrition and alternative/complementary therapies for people infected with HIV. This is the revised 6th edittion of *Aids Control Diet* available from Keep Hope Alive (address on page 221).

Lee, William H., *Getting the Best out of Your Juicer* (New Canaan, Conn: Keats Publishing, 1992). A comprehensive book on fruit and vegetable juicing, including recipes and formulas for specific health problems. Widely available.

Passwater, Richard A., *Cancer Prevention and Nutritional Therapies* (New Canaan, Conn: Keats Publishing, 1993). How diet and nutrition can affect the course of cancer.

Robbins, John, *Diet for a New America* (Walpole, N.H.: Stillpoint Publishing, 1987). A well-researched guide to eating low on the food chain.

Shannon, Sara, *Good Health in a Toxic World* (New York: Warner Books,

1994). A comprehensive and well-researched guide to fighting free radicals. Includes exercises and recipes.

Vogel, Alfred, *The Nature Doctor* (New Canaan, Conn: Keats Publishing, 1992). A comprehensive manual on traditional and complementary medicine by a ninety-year-old naturopath. Widely available.

Walker, N. W., *Diet and Salad Suggestions* (Phoenix: Norwalk Press, 1970). A classic raw-foods recipe book, first published in 1940.

Walker, N. W., *Raw Vegetable Juices* (New York: Jove Books, 1989). This is a reprint of Walker's classic, first published in 1936. It is considered the bible on vegetable juicing. Widely available.

Wigmore, Ann, *Overcoming AIDS* (Boston: Ann Wigmore Foundation, 1987). A holistic protocol for AIDS, focusing on body cleansing, living-foods nutrition, and natural rejuvenation. Wigmore wrote many other books on the living-foods lifestyle, sprouting, wheat grass, and related subjects. Available at natural-food stores or from the Ann Wigmore Foundation (address on page 221). Other information about Ann Wigmore's approach to healing can be found in her book *Be Your Own Doctor* (Garden City Park, N.Y.: Avery Books, 1990).

Some General Books on Holistic Health

Anderson, Robert A., *Wellness Medicine* (New Canaan, Conn: Keats Publishing, 1987). A comprehensive, well-researched, and practical guide to health and healing.

Barash, Marc Alan, *The Healing Path* (Los Angeles: Jeremy P. Tarcher, 1993). A self-help book about how "the darkest passage of human life can become a journey to the soul."

Chopra, Deepak, *Quantum Healing* (New York: Bantam New Age, 1989). Exploring the frontiers of mind–body medicine by the well-known holistic physician.

Dethlefsen, Thorwald, and Rudiger Dalhke, *The Healing Power of Illness* (Rockport Mass: Element Books, 1990). A provocative book on the inner meaning of disease symptoms and their psychological interpretations.

Epstein, Donald, with Nathaniel Altman, *The Twelve Stages of Healing* (San Rafael, Calif.: New World Library, 1994). A powerful self-help guide for achieving healing and personal transformation by traveling along the twelve stages of the healing process.

Harrison, John, *Love Your Disease* (Santa Monica, Calif.: Hay House, 1989). A powerful book by a medical doctor that discusses the psychological basis for disease, including information on why people decide to become ill, what we do to prevent recovery, and how self-healing can take place.

Hay, Louise L., *The AIDS Book* (Santa Monica, Calif.: Hay House, 1988). A self-help manual to assist people facing AIDS and other life-threatening illnesses using practical approaches for self-love and personal transformation. Her popular book *You Can Heal Your Life* is also a valuable resource.

Justice, Blair, *Who Gets Sick?* (Los Angeles: Jeremy P. Tarcher, 1988). A comprehensive and well-documented book about how our beliefs, moods, and thoughts affect our health.

Kunz, Dora, ed., *Spiritual Aspects of the Healing Arts* (Wheaton, Ill.: Quest Books, 1985). An excellent anthology exploring many of the deeper aspects of healing from a variety of noted healers.

Locke, Steven, and Douglas Colligan, *The Healer Within* (New York: Mentor Books, 1986). A book about psychoneuroimmunity and mind–body medicine.

Mikluscak-Cooper, Cindy, and Emmett E. Miller, *Living in Hope* (Berkeley: Celestial Arts, 1991). A valuable twelve-step book for people who are at risk of or infected with HIV.

Ornstein, Robert, and David Sobel, *The Healing Brain* (New York: Touchstone, 1989). How the brain can keep us healthy.

Siegel, Bernie S., *Peace, Love and Healing* (New York: Harper-Collins, 1989). An inspiring book about the body–mind connection and the path to self-healing.

Simonton, O. Carl, and Reid Henson, with Brenda Hampton, *The Healing Journey* (New York: Bantam Books, 1992). A mind–body healing book about a cancer patient's experience. Includes exercises in guided imagery and a two-year health plan.

Simonton, O. Carl, Stephanie Mathews-Simonton, and James L. Creighton, *Getting Well Again* (New York: Bantam Books, 1981). A book about the "cancer personality" and ways to overcome the disease by changing one's perspectives.

NOTES

Chapter 1. What Are Bio-oxidative Therapies?

1. R. Radel and M. H. Navidi, *Chemistry* (St. Paul: West Publishing, 1990), 441, 445.

2. S. S. Hendler, *The Oxygen Breakthrough* (New York: Pocket Books,1989), 79.

3. M. Barry and M. Cullen, "The Air You Breathe Up There," *Condé Nast Traveller*, December 1993, 110–12.

4. Otto Warburg, *The Prime Cause and Prevention of Cancer* (Wurzburg: K. Triltsch, 1966).

5. D. M. Considine, ed., *Van Nostrand's Scientific Encyclopedia*, 7th ed., vol. 2 (New York: Van Nostrand Reinhold, 1989), 2112.

6. Natalie Angier, "The Price We Pay for Breathing," *The New York Times Magazine* (April 25, 1993): 64.

7. David Lin, *Free Radicals and Disease Prevention* (New Canaan, Conn: Keats Publishing, 1993), 19–21.

8. Sara Shannon, *Good Health in a Toxic World: The Complete Guide to Fighting Free Radicals* (New York: Warner Books, 1994).

9. Stephen A. Levine and Parris M. Kidd, *Antioxidant Adaptation* (San Leandro, Calif.: Allergy Research Group, 1986), 63.

10. Angier, op. cit., 100.

11. Marie Thérès Jacobs, "Adverse Effects and Typical Complications in Ozone–Oxygen Therapy," *Ozonachrichten* 1 (1982): 193–201.

12. I. N. Love, "Peroxide of Hydrogen as a Remedial Agent," *Journal of the American Medical Association* (March 3, 1888): 262–265

13. Pamela S. Grim et al., "Hyperbaric Oxygen Therapy," *Journal of the American Medical Association* (April 25, 1990): 2216.

14. *Oxidative Therapy* (Oklahoma City: International Bio-Oxidative Medicine Foundation, n.d.), 2–3.

15. Frank Shallenberger, "Intravenous Ozone Therapy in HIV Related Disease," *Proceedings: Fourth International Bio-Oxidative Medical Conference* (April 1993).

16. Robert Atkins, interview in *Ozone and the Politics of Medicine* (Vancouver: Threshold Film, 1993).

17. M. T. Carpendale, interview in *Ozone and the Politics of Medicine* (Vancouver: Threshold Film, 1993).

18. Horst Kief, interview in *Ozone and the Politics of Medicine* (Vancouver: Threshold Film, 1993).

19. *The Value Line Investment Survey*, 8th ed., Part 3 (August 1, 1997) 1236.

Chapter 2. Ozone

1. *Chemical Technology: An Encyclopedic Treatment*, vol. 1 (New York: Barnes & Noble, 1968), 79.

2. Siegfried Rilling and Renate Viebahn, *The Use of Ozone in Medicine* (Heidelberg: Haug Publishers, 1987), 17.

3. A. C. Baggs, "Are Worry-Free Transfusions Just a Whiff of Ozone Away?" *Canadian Medical Association Journal* (April 1, 1993): 1159.

4. Margaret Gilpin, "Update-Cuba: On the Road to a Family Medicine Nation," *Journal of Public Health Policy* 12, no. 1 (spring 1991): 90–91.

5. Andrés Oppenheimer, *Castro's Final Hour* (New York: Touchstone Books, 1993), 82–83.

6. *Chemical Technology*, op. cit., pp. 82–83.

7. *McGraw-Hill Encyclopedia of Science & Technology*, 6th ed., vol. 12 (New York: McGraw-Hill, 1987), 610.

8. Othmer, *Encyclopedia of Chemical Technology*, 3rd ed., vol. 16 (New York: John Wiley & Sons, 1981), 705.

9. Ibid., 704.

10. James Dulley, "The Sensible Home: Ozone Is a Solid Pool, Spa Purifier," *Los Angeles Times* Home Edition, Real Estate (May 12, 1996): 5.

11. *Chemical Technology*, op. cit., 82.

12. Othmer, op. cit., 710.

13. See notes 11 and 12 above.

14. Rilling and Viebahn, op. cit.,17.

15. Ibid., 177–78; *Proceedings of the First Iberolatinamerican Congress on Ozone*

Application (Havana: National Center for Scientific Research, 1990); *Revista CENIC Ciencias Biológicas*, 20, no. 1–2–3, (1989); Silvia Menéndez, *Ozomed/Ozone Therapy* (Havana: National Center for Scientific Research, 1993).

16. Fritz Kramer, "Ozone in the Dental Practice," in *Medical Applications of Ozone*, edited by Julius LaRaus (Norwalk, Conn: International Ozone Association, Pan American Committee, 1983), 258–65.

17. Gerard Sunnen, "Ozone in Medicine: Overview and Future Direction," *Journal of Advancement in Medicine* 1, no. 3 (fall 1988).

18. Rilling and Viebahn, op. cit., 136–37.

19. Horst Kief, *Therapeutic Significance of Intestinal Insufflation of Medical Ozone*, monograph (Ludwigshafen: Kief Clinic, n.d.).

20. *Proceedings of the First Iberolatinamerican Congress*, op. cit.

21. V. Bocci, "Ozonetherapy Today," in *Ozone in Medicine: Proceedings 12th World Congress of the International Ozone Association* (Zurich: International Ozone Association, 1995), 14.

22. Sunnen, op. cit.

23. S. N. Gorbunov et al., "The Use of Ozone in the Treatment of Children Suffered Due to Different Catastrophies," in *Ozone in Medicine: Proceedings 11th Ozone World Congress* (Stamford, Conn.: International Ozone Association, Pan American Committee, 1993), M–3–31–33.

24. Horst Kief, *The Autohomologous Immune Therapy*, monograph, (Ludwigshafen: Kief Clinic, 1992).

Chapter 3. Hydrogen Peroxide

1. Ed McCabe, *O$_2$xygen Therapies* (Morrisville, N.Y.: Energy Publications, 1988), 24–25.

2. Anthony di Fabio, *Supplement to the Art of Getting Well,* chap. 3 (Franklin, Tenn.: The Rheumatoid Disease Foundation, 1989), 17.

3. C. H. Farr, *Protocol for the Intravenous Administration of Hydrogen Peroxide* (Oklahoma City: International Bio-Oxidative Medicine Foundation, 1993), 29–31.

4. *McGraw-Hill Encyclopedia of Science and Technology*, 6th ed., vol. 12 (New York: McGraw-Hill, 1987), 596.

5. Letter from Randall Prue to Oxytherapy.com, March 15, 1996.

6. *Hydrogen Peroxide Uses in Agriculture* (Glencoe, Minn.: Farmgard Products, n.d.).

7. I. N. Love, "Peroxide of Hydrogen as a Remedial Agent," *Journal of the American Medical Association* (March 3, 1888): 262–65.

8. P. R. Cortelyou, "80 Years Ago: Use of Peroxide of Hydrogen in Diseases of the Throat and Nose," *Journal of the Medical Association of Georgia* (September 1968): 449–50 [the original article appeared in 1888].

9. T. H. Oliver and D. V. Murphy, "Influenzal Pneumonia: The Intravenous Use of Hydrogen Peroxide," *The Lancet,* February 21, 1920, 432–33.

10. McCabe, op. cit., 148–49.

11. J. W. Finney et al., "Protection of the Ischemic Heart with DMSO Alone or DMSO with Hydrogen Peroxide," *Annals of the New York Academy of Sciences* 151 (1967): 231–41.

12. H. C. Urschel Jr., *Circulation* 31, supplement 2 (1965): 203–10.

13. H. C. Urschel Jr., "Cardiovascular Effects of Hydrogen Peroxide," *Diseases of the Chest* 51 (February 1967): 187–88.

14. Farr, op. cit., 32.

15. Ibid., 38–39.

16. di Fabio, op. cit., 15.

17. *Oxidative Therapy* (Oklahoma City: International Bio-Oxidative Medicine Foundation, n.d.), 3.

18. Betsy Russel-Manning, ed., *Self-Treatment for AIDS, Oxygen Therapies, etc.* (San Francisco: Greensward Press, 1988), 19.

19. Kurt Donsbach, *Oxygen–Peroxides–Ozone* (Tulsa: Rockland Corporation, 1993), 44–45.

20. Conrad LeBeau, *Hydrogen Peroxide Therapy,* 9th ed. (Monterey, Calif.: Conrad LeBeau, 1993), 8–9.

21. Donsbach, op. cit., 45.

22. Communication from Charles H. Farr, February 4, 1994.

23. Y. Oya et al., "The Biological Activity of Hydrogen Peroxide," *Mutation Research* 172 (1986): 245–53.

24. Bill Thomson, "Do Oxygen Therapies Work?" *East West* (September 1989): 110.

25. C. H. Farr, "The Use of Hydrogen Peroxide to Inject Trigger Points, Soft Tissue Injuries and Inflamed Joints," monograph (Oklahoma City: C. H. Farr, 1993).

26. Farr, *Protocol,* op. cit., 9–13.

PART II. BIO-OXIDATIVE THERAPIES IN MEDICINE

1. J. Varro, "Ozone Applications in Cancer Cases," in *Medical Applications of Ozone,* edited by Julius LaRaus (Norwalk, Conn.: International Ozone Association, Pan American Committee, 1983), 98.

2. Paul A. Sergios, *One Boy at War: My Life in the AIDS Underground* (New York: Alfred A. Knopf, 1993), 84.

3. Ibid.

4. Sheryl Gay Stolberg, "U.S. AIDS Research Abroad Sets off Outcry over Ethics," *The New York Times* (September 18, 1997): A1.

Chapter 4. Cardiovascular Disease

1. Davor Huic, "Nicaragua's Ortega in Cuba for Medical Check," Reuters, February 1, 1996.
2. Siegfried Rilling and Renate Viebahn, *The Use of Ozone in Medicine* (Heidelberg: Haug Publishers, 1987), 48.
3. R. T. Canoso et al., "Hydrogen Peroxide and Platelet Function," *Blood* 43, no. 5 (May 1974).
4. B. N. Yamaja Setty et al., "Effects of Hydrogen Peroxide on Vascular Arachidonic Acid Metabolism," *Prostaglandins Leukotrienes and Medicine* 14 (1984): 205–13; P. H. Levine et al., "Leukocyte-Platelet Interaction," *Journal of Clinical Investigation* 57 (April 1976): 955–63.
5. C. H. Farr, "The Therapeutic Use of Hydrogen Peroxide," *Townsend Letter for Doctors* (July 1987): 185.
6. R. Viebahn, "The Biochemical Processes Underlying Ozone Therapy," *OzoNachrichten* Heft 1/2 (January 4, 1985).
7. N. I. Zhulina et al., "Ozonotherapy Efficiency in the Treatment of Patients with Atherosclerosis of Coronary and Cerebral Vessels," *Ozone in Medicine: Proceedings of the Eleventh Ozone World Congress* (Stamford, Conn.: International Ozone Association, Pan American Committee, 1993), M–2–9–11.
8. Frank Hernández, et al., "Decrease of Blood Cholesterol and Stimulation of Antioxidative Response in Cardiopathy Patients Treated with Endovenous Ozone Therapy," *Free Radical Biology and Medicine* (July 1995): 115–19.
9. G. Verrazzo, et al., "Hyperbaric Oxygen, Oxygen–Ozone Therapy, and Rheologic Parameters of Blood in Patients with Peripheral Occlusive Arterial Disease." *Undersea Hyberbaric Medicine* (March 1995): 17–22.
10. Ottokar Rokitansky, "Clinical Study of Ozone Therapy in Peripheral Arterial Circulatory Disorders," in *Medical Applications of Ozone*, edited by Julius LaRaus (Norwalk, Conn.: International Ozone Association, Pan American Committee, 1983), 33–54.
11. A. Romero et al., "La ozonoterapia en la aterosclerosis obliterante," *Revista CENIC Ciencias Biológicas* 20, no. 1–2–3: 70–76.
12. J. Sroczynski et al., "[Various Parameters of Lipid Metabolism after Intraarterial Injections of Ozone in Patients with Ischemia of the Lower Extremities and Diabetes Mellitus]," *Polski Tygodnik Lekarski* (November 19–26, 1990): 953–55 [in Polish].
13. B.Turczynski et al., "[Ozone Therapy and Viscosity of Blood and Plasma, Distance of Intermittent Claudication and Certain Biochemical Plasma Components in Patients with Occlusive Arteriosclerosis of the Lower Limbs]," *Polski Tygodnik Lekarski* (September 9–30, 1991): 700–703 [in Polish].

14. J. Sroczynski et al., "[Clinical Assessment of Treatment Results for Athero-sclerotic Ischemia of the Lower Extremities with Intra-arterial Ozone Injections]," *Polski Tygodnik Lekarski* (October 19, 1992): 964–66 [in Polish].

15. S. N Gorbudnov et al., "Medical Ozone in the Treatment of Lower Extremities Peripheral Circulation Disorders," in *Proceedings: Ozone in Medicine, 12th World Congress of the International Ozone Association* (Zurich: International Ozone Association, 1995), 109–110.

16. A. Romero, et al., "Arteriosclerosis Obliterans and Ozone Therapy: Its administration by Different Routes," *Angiologia* (September–October 1993): 177–79.

17. B. A. Korolyov et al., "Ozone Application by Cardiosurgical Patients in Correction of Heart Defects, Complicated by Infectious Endocarditis," *Ozone in Biology and Medicine* (Nizhni Novgorod: Ministry of Public Health of Russia Federation, 1992), 88.

18. J. W. Finney et al., "Removal of Cholesterol and Other Lipids from Experimental Animal and Human Atheromatous Arteries by Dilute Hydrogen Peroxide," *Proceedings: in 3rd International Symposium on Hyperbaric Medicine* (1965).

19. F. Hernández et al., "Effect of Endovenous Ozone Therapy on Lipid Pattern and Antioxidative Response of Ischemia Cardiopathy Patients," *in Ozone in Medicine: Proceedings of the 11th Ozone World Congress* (Stamford, Conn.: International Ozone Association, Pan American Committee, 1993), M–2–12–19.

20. H. C. Urschel Jr., "Cardiovascular Effects of Hydrogen Peroxide," *Diseases of the Chest* 51 (February 1967): 187–88.

21. J. W. Finney et al., "Protection of the Ischemic Myocardium with DMSO Alone or in Combination with Hydrogen Peroxide," *Annals New York Academy of Sciences* (1967).

22. Y. Shaarov et al., "Ozone Therapy in Ischemic Heart Disease (IHD)," in *Abstracts: 2nd International Symposium on Ozone Applications* (Havana: Ozone Research Center, 1997), 56–57.

23. S. P. Peretyagin, "Mechanisms of Ozone Medicinal Effect in Case of Hypoxy," *Ozone in Biology and Medicine* (Nizhni Novgorod: Ministry of Public Health of Russia Federation, 1992), 76.

24. E. Devesa et al., "Ozone Therapy in Ischemic Cerebro-vascular Disease," in *Ozone in Medicine: Proceedings of the 11th Ozone World Congress* (Stamford, Conn.: International Ozone Association, Pan American Committee, 1993), M–4–10–18.

25. Gerd Wasser, "Additional Therapy of Cerebro-vascular Disorder (here: Acute Brain Stroke) by Ozone Therapy," in *Proceedings: Ozone in Medicine, 12th World Congress of the International Ozone Association* (Zurich: International Ozone Association, 1995), 91–95.

Chapter 5. Cancer

1. Otto Warburg, *The Prime Cause and Prevention of Cancer* (Wurzburg: K Tritsch, 1966).
2. James D. Watson, *Molecular Biology of the Gene* (New York: W. A. Benjamin, 1965), 469.
3. J. Varro, "Die krebsbehandlung mit ozon," *Erfahrungsheilkunde* 23 (1974): 178–81.
4. F. Sweet et al., "Ozone Selectively Inhibits Growth of Cancer Cells," *Science* 209 (August 22, 1980): 931–32.
5. Betsy Russell-Manning, ed., *Self-Treatment for AIDS: Oxygen Therapies* (San Francisco: Greenwood Press; 1988), 23.
6. J. T. Mallams et al., "The Use of Hydrogen Peroxide as a Source of Oxygen in a Regional Intra-arterial Infusion System," *Southern Medical Journal* (March 1962).
7. B. L. Aronoff et al., "Regional Oxygenation in Neoplasms," *Cancer* 18 (October 1965): 1250.
8. H. Sasaki et al., "Application of Hydrogen Peroxide to Maxillary Cancer," *Yonago Acta Medica* 11, no. 3 (1967): 149.
9. C. F. Nathan, and Z. A. Cohn, "Antitumor Effects of Hydrogen Peroxide in Vivo," *Journal of Experimental Medicine* 154 (November 1981): 1548.
10. C. F. Nathan et al., "Extracellular Cytolysis by Activated Macrophages and Granulocytes," *Journal of Experimental Medicine* 149 (January 1979): 109.
11. M. K. Samoszuk et al., "In Vitro Sensitivity of Hodgkin's Disease to Hydrogen Peroxide Toxicity," *Cancer* 63 (1989): 2114.
12. M. Arnan, and L. E. DeVries, "Effect of Ozone/Oxygen Gas Mixture Directly Injected into the Mammary Carcinoma of the Female C3H/HEJ Mice," in *Medical Applications of Ozone*, edited by Julius LaRaus (Norwalk, Conn.: International Ozone Association Pan American Committee, 1983), 101–7.
13. L. Paulesu et al., "Studies on the Biological Effects of Ozone, 2, Induction of Tumor Necrosis Factor on Human Leucocytes," *Lymphokine and Cytokine Research* 10, no. 5 (1991): 409–12.
14. Sweet, op. cit.
15. J. Varro, in "Ozone Applications in Cancer Cases," *Medical Applications of Ozone*, edited by Julius LaRaus (Norwalk, Conn.: International Ozone Association Pan American Committee, 1983), 94–95.
16. Ibid., 97–98.
17. Kurt W. Donsbach, and H. R. Alsleben, *Wholistic Cancer Therapy* (Tulsa: Rockland Corporation, 1992), 49.
18. Kurt W. Donsbach *Oxygen–Peroxides-Ozone*, 66.
19. Letter from Dr. Kurt W. Donsbach, December 30, 1993.

20. Interview with Jon Greenberg, M.D., December 21, 1993.
21. Interview with Horst Kief, M.D., December 15, 1993.
22. Ibid.
23. Carl Franklin, "Oxygen Is Key to Tumor Treatment," *New Scientist* (May 7 1994): 17.

Chapter 6. HIV/AIDS

1. Unpublished data, Division of PHS Budget, U.S. Public Health Service, Dept. of Health and Human Services, Bethesda, Md. (April 22, 1994), 5.
2. Burroughs Wellcome Financial Report, 1992–1993.
3. Siegfried Rilling and Renate Viebahn, *The Use of Ozone in Medicine* (Heidelberg: Haug Publishers, 1987), 41–44.
4. "HIV Clue Announced," *American Medical News* (March 1, 1993): 25.
5. *CDC National AIDS Hotline Training Bulletin*, no. 67 (November 31, 1993), 1.
6. UNAIDS/WHO Working Group on Global HIV/AIDS and STD Surveillance, "Report on the Global HIV/AIDS Eppidemic," (November 27, 1997) 2.
7. Peter Duisberg, "HIV and AIDS: Correlation but Not Causation," *Proceedings of the New York Academy of Sciences* 86 (February 1989): 755–64.
8. *Health Facts* (July 1992): 4.
9. Ibid.
10. Interview with Dr. Juliane Sacher, January 26, 1994.
11. Letter from Dr. Frank Shallenberger, December 9, 1993.
12. M. T. Carpendale and J. K. Freeberg, "Ozone Inactivates HIV at Non-Cytotoxic Concentrations," *Antiviral Research* 16 (1991): 281–92.
13. K. H. Wells et al., "Inactivation of Human Immunodeficiency Virus Type I by Ozone In Vitro," *Blood* 78, no. 7 (October 1, 1991): 1882.
14. G. V. Kornilaeva et al., "Ozone Influence on HIV Infection in Vitro," *Ozone in Biology and Medicine* (Nizhni Novgorod: Ministry of Public Health of Russia Federation, 1992), 86.
15. A. C. Baggs, "Are Worry-Free Transfusions Just a Whiff of Ozone Away?" *Canadian Medical Association Journal* (April 1, 1993): 1159.
16. M. E. Shannon, interview in *Ozone and the Politics of Medicine* (Vancouver: Threshold Film, 1993).
17. Horst Kief, "Die Biologischen Grundlagen der Autohomologen Immunotherapie," *Erfahrungsheilkunde* 37, no. 7 (July 1988): 175–80.
18. Horst Kief, interview in *Ozone and the Politics of Medicine* (Vancouver: Threshold Film, 1993).
19. Alexander Pruess, "Positive Treatment Results in AIDS Therapy," *OzoNachrichten* 5 (1986): 3–5.

20. Horst Kief, *Ozone and the Auto-homologous Immune Therapy in AIDS Patients*, monograph (Ludwigshafen: Kief Clinic, 1993).
21. M. T. Carpendale and J. Griffiss, "Is There a Role for Medical Ozone in the Treatment of HIV and Associated Infections?" in *Ozone in Medicine: Proceedings of the 11th Ozone World Congress* (Stamford, Conn.: International Ozone Association, Pan American Committee, 1993), M–1–38–43.
22. M. T. Carpendale et al., "Does Ozone Alleviate AIDS Diarrhea?" *Journal of Clinical Gastroenterology* 17 (1993): 142–45.
23. F. Shallenberger, "Intravenous Ozone Therapy in HIV-Related Disease," in *Proceedings: 4th International Bio-Oxidative Medicine Conference* (Oklahoma City: IBOM, 1993).
24. Case Studies, Monograph (Salisbury, N.C.: Cure AIDS Now, 1993).
25. John C. Pittman,"Introduction," monograph (Salisbury, N.C.: Cure AIDS Now, 1993), 2.
26. G. E. Garber et al., "The Use of Ozone Treated Blood in the Therapy of HIV Infection and Immune Disease," *AIDS* 5 (1991): 981–84.
27. Letter from Capt. Michael E. Shannon, January 21, 1994.
28. Letter from Dr. M. E. Shannon to Ed McCabe, January 13, 1995.
29. Interview with Dr. Silvia Menéndez, January 6, 1994.
30. *A Special Report from Keep Hope Alive*, no. 4 (December 13, 1993), 2.
31. M. T. Carpendale and J. Griffiss, "Is there a Role for Medical Ozone in the Treatment of HIV and Associated Infections?" in *Ozone in Medicine: Proceedings of the 11th Ozone World Congress* (Stamford, Conn.: International Ozone Association, Pan American Committee, 1993), M–1–38.
32. Mark Konlee, *AIDS Control Diet*, 4th ed. (W. Allis, Wisc.: Keep Hope Alive, 1992), 36–37 [revised and retitled *How to Reverse Immune Dysfunction*].
33. Statement by Randolph F. Wykoff before the Committee on the Judiciary, Subcommittee on Crime and Criminal Justice, House of Representatives, (May 23, 1993).
34. Testimony by Richard Schrader on AIDS Fraud before the Committee on the Judiciary, Subcommittee on Crime and Criminal Justice, House of Representatives, (May 23, 1993).

Chapter 7. Additional Applications of Bio-oxidative Therapies

1. Jon Greenberg, "An Auto-vaccine for Human Use Produced with the Aid of Ozone Gas," *in Ozone in Medicine: Proceedings of the 11th Ozone World Congress* (Stamford, Conn.: International Ozone Association, Pan American Committee, 1993), M–3–21.
2. Capt. M. E. Shannon interview in "Ozone and the Politics of Medicine" (Vancouver: Threshold Film, 1993).

3. *Proceedings of the Tenth Ozone World Congress* (Monaco, 1991), 87–93.

4. R. Wong et al., "Ozonoterapia analgésica," *Revista CENIC Ciencias Biológicas* 20 (1989): 143.

5. E. Riva Sanseverino, "Knee-Joint Disorders Treated by Oxygen–Ozone Therapy," *Europa Medicophysica* 25, no. 3 (1989): 163–70.

6. Gilbert Glady, "Diverse Pathology Treated in Medical Ozone Clinic," in *Ozone in Medicine: Proceedings of the 11thOzone World Congress* (Stamford, Conn.: International Ozone Association, Pan American Committee, 1993), M–3–3.

7. H. Kief, "Die Behandlung des Asthma bronchiale mit der autohomologen Immuntherapie (AHIT)," *Erfahrungsheilkunde* 9 (1990): 534.

8. J. Ramos et al., "Estudio imunológico de 25 pacientes grandes quemados tratados con ozono," *Revista CENIC Ciencias Biológicas* 20, no. 1–2–3: 116–20.

9. C. H. Farr, *The Therapeutic Use of Intravenous Hydrogen Peroxide*, monograph (Oklahoma City: Genesis Medical Center, January 1987), 18–19.

10. N. Velasco, "Valor de la ozonoterapia en el tratamiento del pie diabético neuroinfeccioso," *Revista CENIC Ciencias Biológicas* 20, no. 1–2–3: 64–70.

11. E. Pavlovskaya et al., "Effectiveness of Ozone Therapy in the Process of Diabetes Treatment," in *Abstracts: 2nd International Symposium on Ozone Applications* (Havana: Ozone Research Center/National Center for Scientific Research, 1997), 50.

12. R. Behar et al., "Tratamiento de la úlcera gastrodoudenal con ozono," *Revista CENIC Ciencias Biológicas* 20, no. 1–2–3: 60–61.

13. A. Gierek-Lapinska et al., "Preliminary Report on Using General Ozone Therapy in Diseases of the Posterior Segment of the Eye," *Klin. Oszna* (May–June 1992):139–40.

14. Silvia Menéndez et al., "Ozone Therapy and Magneto Therapy: New Methods for the Rehabilitation of Patients with Simple Chronic Glaucoma," in *Proceedings: Ozone in Medicine, 12th World Congress of the International Ozone Association* (Zurich: International Ozone Association, 1995), 99–106.

15. R. Santiesteban et al., "Ozone Therapy in Optic Nerve Dysfunction," in *Ozone in Medicine: Proceedings of the Eleventh Ozone World Congress* (Stamford, Conn.: International Ozone Association, Pan American Committee, 1993), M–4–1–9.

16. R. Santiesteban, et al., "Ozone Therapy in Patients Suffering from Optic Nerve Dysfunction," in *Abstracts: 2nd International Symposium on Ozone Applications* (Havana: Ozone Research Center/National Center for Scientific Research, 1997), 40.

17. E. Riva Sanseverino et al., "Effects of Oxygen–Ozone Therapy on Age-Related Degenerative Retinal Maculopathy," *Panminerva Medica* (April–June 1990): 77–84.

18. S. Menéndez et al., "Aplicación de la ozonoterapia en la retinosis pigmentaria," *Revista CENIC Ciencias Biológicas* 20, no. 1–2–3: 84–90.

19. E. C. Diaz et al., "Ozone Therapy in Different Ophthalmologic Diseases," in *Abstracts: 2nd International Symposium on Ozone Applications* (Havana: Ozone Research center/ National Center for Scientific Research, 1997), 38–39.

20. M. Copello et al., "Ten Year Study in Patients Suffering from Retinitis Pigmentosa and Treated with Repeated Cycles of Ozone Therapy," in *Abstracts: 2nd International Symposium on Ozone Applications* (Havana: Ozone Research Center/National Center for Scientific Research, 1997), 36.

21. Interview with Rosaralis Santiesteban, M.D., January 5, 1994.

22 R. A. Mayer, "Experiences of a Pediatrician Using Ozone as a Chemotherapeutic Agent for the Treatment of Diseases of Children," in *Medical Applications of Ozone*, edited by Julius LaRaus (Norwalk, Conn.: International Ozone Association, Pan American Committee, 1983), 210.

23. J. O. Sardina et al., "Tratamiento de la giardiasis recidivante con ozono," *Revista CENIC Ciencias Biológicas* 20, no. 1–2–3: 61–64.

24. Silvia Menéndez et al., "Application of Ozonized Oil in the Treatment of Infantile Giardiasis," in *Proceedings: Ozone in Medicine, 12th World Congress of the International Ozone Association* (Zurich: International Ozone Association, 1995), 297–300.

25. T. de las Cagigas et al., "Use of Ozonized Oil on Patients with Vulvovaginitis," *First Iberolatinamerican Congress on Ozone Applications* (Havana: National Center for Scientific Research, 1990), 66.

26. T. S. Kachalina et al., "Some Aspects of Ozone Therapy Application in Gynecological Practice," in *Ozone in Biology and Medicine* (Nizhni Novgorod: Ministry of Public Health of Russia Federation, 1992), 90.

27. N. M. Pobedinsky et al., "Effectiveness of Ozone Therapy in the Treatment of Condilomatosis in Women," *Ozone in Biology and Medicine* (Nizhni Novgorod: Ministry of Public Health of Russia Federation, 1992), 90.

28. Ernesto Basabe et al., "Ozone Therapy Like a Favoring Element in the Rehabilitation of Children with Hearing Loss," in *Proceedings: Ozone in Medicine, 12th World Congress of the International Ozone Association* (Zurich: International Ozone Association, 1995), 275–78.

29. H. Konrad, "Ozone vs. Hepatitis and Herpes," in *Medical Applications of Ozone*, edited by Julius LaRaus (Norwalk, Conn., International Ozone Association, Pan American Committee, 1983), 140–41.

30. Y. Betancourt et al., "Ozone Therapy: A Useful Alternative on Virulent Hepatitis Treatment," in *Abstracts: 2nd International Symposium on Ozone Applications* (Havana: Ozone Research Center, 1997), 61–62.

31. Ronald M. Davis, M.D., monograph, 5002 Todville, Seabrook, TX 77586.

32. Silvia Menéndez et al., "Application of Ozone Therapy in Children with Humoral Immunity Deficiency," in *Proceedings: Ozone in Medicine, 12th World Congress of the International Ozone Association* (Zurich: International Ozone Association, 1995), 271–74.

33. C. H. Farr, "Rapid Recovery from Type A/Shanghai Influenza Treated with Intravenous Hydrogen Peroxide," monograph (Oklahoma City: C. H. Farr, 1993).

34. Kenneth Bock, "Oxidative Modalities in Lyme Disease," talk at the 8th International Bio-Oxidative Conference, Anchorage, Alaska (May 18, 1997).

35. H. M. Dockrell and H. L. Playfair, "Killing of Blood-Stage Murine Malaria Parasites by Hydrogen Peroxide," *Infection and Immunity* (January 1983): 456–59.

36. G. O. Grechkanyov and T. S. Kachalaina, "Ozone Therapy in a Complex Treatment of Threatened Abortion," in *Proceedings: Ozone in Medicine, 12th World Congress of the International Ozone Association* (Zurich: International Ozone Association, 1995), 291–94.

37. J. Wennstrom and J. Lindhe, "Effect of Hydrogen Peroxide on Developing Plaque and Gingivitis in Man," *Journal of Clinical Periodontology* 6 (1979): 115–30.

38. M. V. Marshall et al., "Hydrogen Peroxide: A Review of Its Use in Dentistry," *Journal of Periodontology* (September 1995): 786–96.

39. G. Klinger et al., "Bacteriological Studies During Conservative Treatment of Periapical Inflammations," *Stomatol-DDR* (December 25, 1975): 801–08.

40. H. Kief, "Die Behandlung der Neurodermatitis mit autohomologer Immuntherapie (AHIT)," *Erfahrungsheilkunde* 1 (1989).

41. H. Kief, "Die Behandlung der Neurodermatitis mit AHIT," *Erfahrungsheilkunde* 3a (March 1993): 166–89.

42. C. H Siemsen, "The Use of Ozone in Orthopedics," in *Proceedings: Ozone in Medicine, 12th World Congress of the International Ozone Association* (Zurich: International Ozone Association, 1995), 125–30.

43. A. Ceballos, "Tratamiento de la osteoartritis con ozono," *Revista CENIC Ciencias Biológicas* 20, no. 1–2–3: 152.

44. E. Riva Sanseverino, "Intensive Medical and Physical Treatment of Osteoporosis with the Aid of Oxygen-Ozone Therapy," *Europa Medicophysica* 24, no. 4 (1988): 199–206.

45. Interview with Dr. Horst Kief, December 15, 1993.

46. M. Rodríguez et al., "Ozone Therapy in the Treatment of Elderly Patients Suffering from Parkinson's Syndromes," in *Abstracts: 2nd International Symposium on Ozone Applications* (Havana: Ozone Research Center/National Center for Scientific Research, 1997), 43–44.

47. I. T. Vasilyev, "Perspectives of Ozone Application in the Treatment of Diffused Peritonitis," *Ozone in Biology and Medicine* (Nizhni Novgorod: Ministry of Public Health of Russia Federation, 1992), 89.

48. E. Riva Sanseverino and P. Castellacci, "Oxygen–Ozone Therapy and Physical Activity in Humans," in *Proceedings: Ozone in Medicine, 12th World Congress of the International Ozone association* (Zurich: International Ozone Association, 1995), 65–72.

49. H. Kawalsky et al., "The Use of Ozonotherapy in Nose Correction Operations," *Acta Chirirgiae Plasticae* 34, 3 (1992): 182–84.

50. F. Menéndez et al., "Ozonoterapia en la artritis reumatoidea," *Revista CENIC Ciencias Biológicas* 20, no. 1–2–3: 144–51.

51. J. Greenberg, "An Auto-Vaccine for Human Use Produced with the Aid of Ozone Gas," in *Ozone in Medicine: Proceedings of the 11th Ozone World Congress* (Stamford, Conn.: International Ozone Association, Pan American Committee, 1993), M–3–21.

52. M. Rodríguez et al., "Ozone Therapy for Senile Dementia," in *Ozone in Medicine: Proceedings of the 11th Ozone World Congress* (Stamford, Conn.: International Ozone Association, Pan American Committee, 1993), M–4–19–25.

53. M. Casas, et al., "Ozone Therapy in Demential Syndrome in the Elderly," in *Abstracts: 2nd International Symposium on Ozone Applications* (Havana: Ozone Research Center/National Center for Scientific Research, 1997), 42–43.

54. Interview with Josué García, M.D., January 6, 1994.

55. H. Calvo et al., "Experiencias preliminares en la utilización del ozono en pacientes de terapia intensiva del hospital 'Carlos J. Finlay'," *Revista CENIC Ciencias Biológicas* 20, no. 1–2–3: 128–35.

56. S. Menéndez et al., "Application of Medical Ozone Therapy in Patients with Sickle Cell Anemia: Preliminary Report," in *Ozone in Medicine: Proceedings of the Eleventh Ozone World Congress* (Stamford, Conn.: International Ozone Association, Pan American Committee, 1993), M–3–12–17.

57. Stephen B. Edelson, *Silicone Immune Dysfunction Syndrome*, monograph (Atlanta: Environmental & Preventive Health Center, 1994).

58. S. L. Krivatkin, "The Experience of Ozone Therapy in Dermato-venereological Dispensary," in *Ozone in Medicine: Proceedings of the 11th Ozone World Congress* (Stamford, Conn.: International Ozone Association, Pan American Committee, 1993), M–3–5–11.

59. S. Krivatkin et al., "Ozonetherapy in Out-patient Dermatological Practice" in *Proceedings: Ozone in Medicine, 12th World Congress of the International Ozone Association* (Zurich: International Ozone Association, 1995), 157–63.

60. T. de las Cagigas et al., "Ozonized Oil and Its Efficacy in Epidermophitosis," *First Iberolatinamerican Congress on Ozone Applications* (Havana: Natural Center for Scientific Research, 1990), 63.

61. Konrad, op. cit., 144.

62. R. Mattassi et al., "Ozone as Therapy in Herpes Simplex and Herpes Zoster Diseases," in *Medical Applications of Ozone*, edited by Julius LaRaus (Norwalk, Conn.: International Ozone Association, Pan American Committee, 1983), 136.

63. Ibid., 134.

64. J. Delgado, "Tratamiento con ozono del herpes zoster," *Revista CENIC Ciencias Biológicas* 20, no. 1–2–3: 160–62.

65. Konrad, op. cit., 147.

66. Heinz Konrad, "Ozone Therapy for Herpes Simplex and Herpes Zoster," in *Proceedings: Ozone in Medicine, 12th World Congress of the International Ozone Association* (Zurich: International Ozone Association, 1995), 189.

67. M. Franzini et al., "Subcutaneous Oxygen–Ozone Therapy in Indurative Hypodermatitis and in Localized Lipodystrophies: A Clinical Study of Efficiency and Tolerability," in *Proceedings: Ozone in Medicine, 12th World Congress of the International Ozone Association* (Zurich: International Ozone Association, 1995), 131–43.

68. Silvia Menéndez et al., "*Onicomycosis Treated with Ozonized Oil*," in *Proceedings: Ozone in Medicine, 12th World Congress of the International Ozone Association* (Zurich: International Ozone Association, 1995), 279–82.

69. M. Manok, "On a Simple and Painless Treatment of Warts," *Hautarzt* 12 (September 1961): 425.

70. Mayer, op. cit., 205.

71. S. N. Gorbunov et al., "The Use of Ozone in the Treatment of Children Suffered Due to Different Catastrophies," in *Ozone in Medicine: Proceedings of the 11th Ozone World Congress* (Stamford, Conn.: International Ozone Association, Pan American Committee, 1993), M–3–31–33.

72. A. A. Priimak et al., "[The Effect of an Ozone–Oxygen Mixture on Mycobacterium Tuberculosis and Conditionally Pathogenic Microorganisms]," *Probl. Tuberk.* 4 (1991): 7–10 [in Russian].

73. T. de las Cagigas et al., "Therapy With Ozonized Oil in Ulcers in Lower Limbs," in *1st Iberolatinamerican Congress on Ozone Applications* (Havana: National Center for Scientific Research, 1990), 64

74. G. A. Balla et. al., "Use of Intra-arterial Hydrogen Peroxide to Promote Wound Healing," *American Journal of Surgery* 108 (November 1964).

PART III. A HOLISTIC PROTOCOL

1. Janet F. Quinn, "The Healing Arts in Modern Health Care," in *Spiritual Aspects of the Healing Arts*, edited by Dora Kunz (Wheaton, Ill: Quest Books, 1985), 121.

2. John C. Pittman, *Comprehensive HIV/AIDS Protocol* (Salisbury, N.C.: Cure AIDS Now, 1993).

Chapter 8. Body Cleansing

1. Robert Gray, *The Colon Health Handbook* (Oakland: Rockridge Publishing, 1982), 29.
2. Horst Kief, "Therapeutic Significance of Intestinal Insufflation of Medical Ozone," monograph (Ludwigshafen: The Kief Clinic, n.d.).
3. Ibid., 37, 44.
4. Max Gerson, *A Cancer Therapy* (Bonita, Calif.: Gerson Institute/Pulse, 1990), 216–17.
5. *Keep Hope Alive Newsletter* (September 27, 1993).
6. Alfred Vogel, *The Nature Doctor* (New Canaan, Conn.: Keats Publishing 1991), 482–83.
7. Interview with Dr. Juliane Sacher, January 26, 1994.

Chapter 9. An Oxygenation Diet

1. David Pimental, *Handbook of Pest Management in Agriculture*, 2nd ed. (Boca Raton, Fla.: CRC Press, 1990).
2. Nathaniel Altman, *Nathaniel Altman's Total Vegetarian Cooking* (New Canaan, Conn.: Keats Publishing, 1980).
3. Sara Shannon, *Good Health in a Toxic World: The Complete Guide to Fighting Free Radicals* (New York: Warner Books 1994), 81.
4. *The New Four Food Groups* (Washington, D.C.: Physicians Committee for Responsible Medicine, 1991).
5. C. H. Farr, *Workbook on Free Radical Chemistry and Hydrogen Peroxide Metabolism* (Oklahoma City, IBOM Foundation, 1993), 46.
6. S. S. Hendler, *The Oxygen Breakthrough* (New York: Pocket Books, 1989), 150.
7. Letter from Dr. Kurt Donsbach, December 30, 1993.
8. Mark Konlee, *AIDS Control Diet*, 6th ed. (W. Allis, Wisc.: Keep Hope Alive, 1994), 68–70.
9. Ann Wigmore, *Overcoming AIDS* (Boston: Ann Wigmore Foundation, 1987), 96.

Chapter 10. Nutritional Supplements and Healing Herbs

1. John C. Pittman, "Comprehensive HIV/AIDS Protocol" (Salisbury, N.C.: Cure AIDS Now, 1993).

2. S. S. Hendler, *The Oxygen Breakthrough* (New York: Pocket Books, 1989), 178.

Chapter 11. Aerobic Exercise and Breathing

1. S. S. Hendler, *The Oxygen Breakthrough* (New York: Pocket Books, 1989), 220.
2. Yogi Ramacharaka, *The Science of Breath* (Chicago: Yogi Publication Society, 1905), 40–41.

Chapter 12. Emotions, Mind, and Spirit

1. Donald Epstein, "There Is No Cure for Healing," *The Network Release* supplement (spring 1993): 1.
2. Larry Dossey, *Space, Time & Medicine* (Boulder: Shambhala Publications, 1982), 183.
3. Sara Shannon, *Good Health in a Toxic World: The Complete Guide to Fighting Free Radicals* (New York: Warner Books, 1994), 180–82.
4. T. Dethlefsen and R. Dahlke, *The Healing Power of Illness* (Rockport, Mass.: Element Books, 1990), 7.
5. O. Carl Simonton, Stephanie Matthews-Simonton, and James L. Creighton, *Getting Well Again* (New York: Bantam Books, 1980), 61–62.
6. Jason Serenus, ed., *Psychoimmunity and the Healing Process* (Berkeley, Calif.: Celestial Arts, 1986), 72.
7. C. Mikluscak-Cooper and E. E. Miller, *Living in Hope* (Berkeley, Calif.: Celestial Arts, 1990), 250.
8. Scott J. Gregory, *A Holistic Protocol for the Immune System* (Joshua Tree, Calif.: Tree of Life Publications, 1989), 83–84.
9. Norman Cousins, *Anatomy of an Illness* (New York: W. W. Norton, 1979).
10. Karen Shultz, "Laughter and Smiling—Good Medicine," in *The Essence of Healing* (Tucson: Theosophical Order of Service, 1984), 62.
11. Louise L. Hay, *The AIDS Book* (Santa Monica, Calif.: Hay House, 1988), 132.
12. Swami Sivananda Radha, *The Divine Light Invocation* (Porthill, Idaho: Timeless Books, 1966).

Chapter 13. Oxygen Products, Services, and Applications

1. Letters from Zdenek Rasplicka of Ozone Services, September 1997.
2. *Code of Federal Regulations—Protection of Environment*, vol. 40, part 50 (Washington, DC: Office of the Federal Register, 1996), 652.

3. Bradford Cook, "Ozone Treatment Gains Popularity," *New Hampshire Business Review*, vol. 18 (May 24, 1996): 19.

4. Letters from Zdenek Rasplicka of Ozone Services, September 1997.

5. Anthony DePalma, "Just When You Thought Air Was Free," *The New York Times* (June 12, 1997): 27, 30.

6. Press release for Oxygen Station, September 1997.

INDEX

nutrition
  AIDS Control Diet, 174–75
  antioxidants, 13–14, 179–83
  diet and diets, 10, 168–77
  detoxification, 158–166
  raw foods, 10, 157, 176–77
  supplements, 157, 178–85
  See also herbs, minerals, vitamins

onicomycosis, 150–51
Oliver, T.H., 50–51, 130
Oppenheimer, Andres, 31
optic atrophy, 119–20
optic nerve dysfunction, 120
Ornstein, Robert, 230
Ortega Saavedra, Daniel, 66
orthopedic problems, 58, 136
OíShaughnessy, Michael, 104
osteoarthritis, 58, 138
osteoporosis, 138–39
oxidation, 11, 14, 15
  definition of, ix–x, 10–11
  oxygen (O_2), 7, 11, 45
  human demands of, 8–9
  deficiency of, x, 11
  bars, 215–16
  products, 216–18
oxygenated water, 216
oxygenation, 157
  and breathing, 191–92
  definition of, x, 11
  diets, 167–77
  and exercise, 187–8
Oxyfresh Worldwide, 225
Oxytherapy.com, 220
ozone (O_3), 7, 11, 24–44, 97–110,
  111–15, 116–29, 130–44,
  145–51, 152–54
  air treatment with, 33–34, 210–12
  dental uses of, 27, 36
  discovery and history of, 26–31
  diseases effective against, 35,
  111–154

generators, 24–25, 27–28, 44,
  209–10
industrial uses of, 33–34
in swimming pools, 32–33, 213–14
in water treatment, 26–27, 32–33,
  213, 214
layer, 24–26
medical uses of, 27–29
resistant materials, 27
toxicity of, 25–26
ozone (O_3) therapies
  autohemotherapy (major and
  minor), 38–39, 40, 65–66, 74–75,
  84, 100
  autohomologous immunotherapy
  (AHIT), 28, 43–44, 87, 98, 114,
  135, 139, 142
  ear insufflation, 41
  inhalation, 42–43
  intra-arterial injection, 37
  intra-articular injection, 39, 70–71
  intramuscular, 33, 94–95, 100
  intravenous injection, 39–41, 148,
  157
  ozonated oil, 42, 147, 149–50,
  152–53
  ozonated water, 39, 125–26,
  151–52, 213, 214
  ozone bagging, 41–42, 60–61,
  116–17
  opposition to, 109–10
  rectal insufflation, 37–38, 77–78,
  86, 100, 108, 123, 142, 144
  steam cabinet method, 41, 163–65
  studies, 83–85, 97–98, 111–54
  See also bio-oxidative therapy
Ozone Services, 44, 160, 164, 211,
  214, 223
Ozonia International, 227

Parkinson's disease, 140
Passwater, Richard A., 228
Pau d'arco, 185